A HANDBOOK FOR MEDICAL ASSISTANTS AND MEDICAL SECRETARIES

A HANDBOOK FOR MEDICAL ASSISTANTS AND MEDICAL SECRETARIES

By

Valeri S. Morimoto, BAE

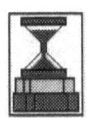

E-BookTime, LLC
Montgomery, Alabama

A HANDBOOK FOR MEDICAL ASSISTANTS AND MEDICAL SECRETARIES

Copyright © 2005 by Valeri S. Morimoto, BAE

All rights reserved. No part of this book may be reproduced or transmitted in any form or by any means, electronic or mechanical, including photocopying, recording, or by any information storage and retrieval system, without permission in writing from the copyright owner.

Library of Congress Control Number: 2005937404

ISBN: 1-59824-096-X

First Edition
Published December 2005
E-BookTime, LLC
6598 Pumpkin Road
Montgomery, AL 36108
www.e-booktime.com

CONTENTS

PREFACE 7
ACKNOWLEDGMENT 9
ABDOMINAL PAIN, VOMITING, DIARRHEA AND
NAUSEA 11
ABO BLOOD GROUPS 12
AMPUTATION 13
ANIMAL BITES 14
ARTERIAL BLOOD GAS (ABG) 15
BACK AND NECK PAIN 16
BLEEDING 17
BLISTERS 18
BLOOD PRESSURE GUIDE 19
BODY MASS INDEX 21
CARDIOVASCULAR PULMONARY RESUSCITATION
(CPR) 23
CHIEF COMPLAINT 24
CHEMICAL BURNS 26
CHOLESTEROL PROFILE (BASIC) 27
CONVERSIONS 28
CPT = Current Procedural Terminology 30
CRUTCHES 31
DEHYDRATION 33
DIABETES MELLITUS (DM) 34
EKG 36
FAINTING 39
FEVER 40
HCPCS ("Hick Picks") 41
HEAD INJURIES 43
HEARING 44
HEAT RELATED EMERGENCIES 45
HEMORRHOIDS 46
ICD-9-CM = International Classification of Diseases 9th
Revision Clinical Modification. 47
IMMUNIZATIONS 49
ABBREVIATIONS 50
INJECTIONS (ID, IM, SQ, Z-track) 51

CONTENTS

INSECT STINGS	55
INTRAVENOUS INFUSION (ASSISTING)	56
LETTERS, MEMOS & CARDS	57
MEDICATION FORMULAS	67
MENTAL STATUS	69
NOSEBLEED	70
PAIN ASSESSMENT	71
PATIENT INTAKE	72
PHYSICAL EXAM	74
POISON (SWALLOWED)	75
PULSE	76
RESPIRATIONS	77
SEA URCHIN SPIKES	78
SEIZURES (CONVULSIONS)	79
SHOCK	80
SKIN CANCER	81
SPRAINS, STRAINS, CONTUSIONS & DISLOCATIONS	82
SUTURES	83
TEMPERATURE CONVERSION	84
THERMAL BURNS	85
TUBERCULIN SKIN TESTING	86
URINARY TRACT INFECTION (UTI)	87
VAGINAL BLEEDING/MISSED PERIOD	88
VENIPUNCTURE	89
WINGED INFUSION OR BUTTERFLY (double-pointed needle) METHOD	92
VISION	93
VITAL SIGN RANGES	94
WEIGHT: (25-99 YEARS OLD)	96
WOUNDS	99
ABBREVIATIONS	101
GLOSSARY	118
BIBLIOGRAPHY	141

PREFACE

Medical Assisting covers a broad field in the healthcare industry. This book is a quick reference for medical assistants and medical secretaries to promote an efficient and well-managed clinic.

ACKNOWLEDGMENT

Special thanks to ABHES Accredited,
Med-Assist School of Hawaii.

ABDOMINAL PAIN, VOMITING, DIARRHEA AND NAUSEA

1. Use the oximeter for O_2 Sat. content.

2. Check to see if vital signs are stable.

3. Check for orthostatic blood pressure by taking the patient's blood pressure in a standing position, sitting position and a supine (lying down) position.

4. If vomiting, provide an emesis basin.

5. Do a dipstick test on a female patient if she has pain, fever, increased frequency, pressure or blood in her urine.

6. Ask female patients for the last menstrual period (LMP) and if she is pregnant. Get a urine specimen if she needs a pregnancy test.

7. Ask the patient if there was blood or the appearance of coffee ground material in vomit and if there has been any blood in the stool or if the stool was black and tarry (Pepto-Bismol may cause this).

8. CAUTION: Some over the counter medicine for diarrhea can worsen certain infections.

ABO BLOOD GROUPS

Blood Type	Antigen present on RBC	Antibody present in Plasma
A	A	B
B	B	A
AB	A, B	None
O	none	A, B

AMPUTATION

If you can find the amputated part (finger, toe, hand or foot), rinse it with sterile or clean water. Wrap it in a clean dressing and place it in a waterproof plastic bag if it fits and place that bag in another container with ice or ice and water. Label the package with the victim's name, date and time. Have it sent to the hospital with the victim. If only a plastic bag and ice is available, rinse and place the body part on top of the ice. Do not submerge it in the cold water. The amputated body part must be saved to be reattached to the person's body.

ANIMAL BITES

1. Apply a cold pack if the skin is not broken.

2. If the skin is broken, wash it with soap and water.

3. Apply direct pressure to control bleeding and seek medical attention.

4. Report domestic animal to the owner if skin is not broken or animal control or police if skin is broken.

5. The animal will be observed for possible rabies.

6. If it is a wild animal, do not try to capture or kill. If you must kill, do not hit or shoot the animal in the brain. Preserve the brain for medical examination by local government health offices.

ARTERIAL BLOOD GAS (ABG)

ABG's are performed to aid in determining metabolic status together with other lab work.

It also helps to determine the patient's present condition. Any abnormality should be reported to an RN or physician. The speed of changes taking place is an important factor in diagnosis and treatment.

pH: serum's acidity, the most important value to assess.

    Acidosis<7.35 -7.45>Alkalosis
               Normal

PO_2: partial pressure of oxygen (Normal 80-100 mmHg)

O_2 Sat: oxygen saturation of blood (Normal 93%)

A hypoxic patient has a low PO_2 and O_2 saturation. Therefore the patient may have inadequate oxygen.

CAUTION: Giving oxygen without knowledge of the exact cause may worsen the patient's condition in such cases as COPD (chronic bronchitis). Notify the RN or physician of any abnormality.

PCO_2 = partial pressure of carbon dioxide (normal 35-45 mmHg)

HCO_3 = bicarbonate serum level (normal 22-28 mEq/L)

BACK AND NECK PAIN

The most common back complaint is in the lower back.

1. Ask if it is in an occupational (job) or a personal injury and record it in the chart. Depending on office policy, you may need to open a separate file for personal injuries or on the job injuries.

2. Do not remove any neck or back brace on the patient and do not move a patient in a wheelchair unless the physician agrees to it or there is proper assistance.

3. If this is a follow up from an ER or hospital visit, ask for records or x-ray reports so the doctor can immediately review them. The transfer of these records often delays the visit.

BLEEDING

1. Locate site of wound and apply direct pressure. Place a sterile dressing or the cleanest cloth available on the wound.

2. Use medical exam gloves if available, extra dressing or plastic wrap.

3. Do not remove an impaled object.

4. If bleeding stops, treat for shock and care for the wound and seek medical attention if necessary.

5. If the bleeding does not stop, raise the extremity above the heart and continue pressing on the wound.

6. If bleeding does not stop, apply pressure and treat for shock.

7. If it does stop, treat for shock and care for wound Seek medical attention if necessary.

8. If bleeding still does not stop, apply tourniquet as a last resort and seek medical attention. Only use a tourniquet in a life or limb situation. Cutting off circulation can lead to amputation.

BLISTERS

Although normally a minor injury, blisters can get infected. If you pop one, leave the top layer of skin on.

1. It is best to leave the blister unbroken.

2. If the pain is unbearable, break the blister by making small holes at the blisters base with a sterile needle.

3. Drain the fluid.

4. Apply a sterile dressing and leave the blisters top on.

5. Watch for signs of infection.

6. If the pain is tolerable, cover the blister with tape, moleskin, doughnut gauze or felt to prevent further injury.

BLOOD PRESSURE GUIDE

1. Ask if there is a history of high blood pressure and the patient's last BP reading.

2. A new patient should have his blood pressure taken on both arms.

3. If you hear the systolic beat immediately, start over again in one minute.

4. Do not say if it is high or low. The physician should explain the results.

Estimated Systolic Pressure

1. Wrap the cuff around the patient's bare arm an inch above the elbow crease. The bladder inside the cuff should cover about 80% of the upper arm in adults and 100% in children. A cuff too large will cause a lower reading and a cuff too small will cause an increased reading.

2. Palpate the radial pulse (thumb side of the wrist) as you inflate the cuff and notice the number the manometer points to when the pulse cannot be felt. This is the estimated systolic pressure.

3. Quickly pump the cuff 20-30 mmHg beyond the estimated systolic pressure.

4. Open the thumbscrew in the "lefty loosey" counter-clockwise direction.

5. Slowly deflate the cuff so the pressure reading falls at 2-3 mmHg per second.

6. Read the manometer when the first sound (systolic) and last sound (diastolic) is heard.

Taking a second BP reading

1. Wait for 1-2 minutes before retaking the reading.

2. Blood stasis may occur from more than 2 readings in the same arm. This will cause an inaccurate reading.

3. Chart the date, time, BP reading and your name.

BODY MASS INDEX

BMI is a method to calculate healthy weight with the measurements of weight in kilograms and height in meters. The equation for a BMI follows.

BMI = kg/meters squared (height x height)

22 pounds = 1 kilogram

(see height and weight)

BMI

<20   underweight
20-25   normal weight
25-30   overweight
30-40   obese
>40   severe obesity

HEIGHT

1 foot = 12 inches
254cm = 1 inch

Example: How many meters is a 5 feet, 4 inch person?
64 inches x 2.54 centimeters = 162.56 cm = 1.63 meters

Example: How many feet is a 1.75 meter patient?

175 m x 3.28 ft/m = 5.74 ft

0.74 ft = 9 inches

12 inches

5 feet + 9 inches = 5'9"

Conversions

1 m = 3.28 ft = 39.37 in
1 cm = 0.4 in = 0.03 ft
1 in = 2.5 cm = 25 mm
1 ft = 12 in = 30.48 cm = 0.3048 m

CARDIOVASCULAR PULMONARY RESUSCITATION (CPR)

	RATE OF COMPRESSIONS	DEPTH OF COMPRESSIONS	RATIO OF COMPRESSIONS (Until signs of circulation)	RESCUE BREATHING (breaths per second)
Adult 2 hands	100/minute or 2/second	1½ to 2 inches	15:2 (four cycles)	1:5
Children (heel of 1 hand)	100/minute or 2/second	1 to 1½ Inches	5:1 Until signs of circulation	1:3
Infants (2 fingers)	100/minute or 2/second	½ to 1 inch (1¼ to 2½ cm)	5:1	1:3

CHIEF COMPLAINT

The main symptom, duration and what the patient has been doing about it.

Watch, listen and ask for the chief complaint. Be concise and use the patient's own words or list the main symptom(s). Observations described in your own words are very important to an emergency caregiver. Watch for signs such as a patient clutching his chest in pain, listen for it realizing that if a patient can't breath, it will stop him from the ability to speak. Remember, only the physician can legally diagnose a patient.

Use open-ended questions for the patient such as "What seems to be the problem today?" or "How may we assist you today?" or "How are you feeling today?" and document the main reason for the visit. An example of documentation is "Pt. c/o of unusual wt loss of 15# during past month." Always believe a patient if he tells you he thinks he is going to die and act on it like it is a true emergency.

Specific Complaints for Prompt Attention

1. Extremely labored, noisy, shallow or absent breathing.

2. Bleeding that is severe or persistent.

3. Pain in the chest, neck, jaw or left arm unrelieved by rest, O_2 or nitrates.

4. Seizures that are prolonged or recurrent, especially if unconscious.

5. Extreme weakness (especially if the patient gets dizzy upon standing).

6. Childbirth close at hand.

7. Headache severe and unrelieved by aspirin or acetaminophen.

8. Abdominal pain that is severe.

9. Palpitations (patient is able to feel heart beating in chest).

10. Extreme trauma (not usually seen in a physician's office)

CHEMICAL BURNS

1. Dry chemicals should be brushed off before washing with water.

2. Wash with water for 20 minutes.

3. Remove clothing and jewelry.

4. Do not try to neutralize and seek medical attention

If it is a caustic wet chemical or corrosive compound such as acid, alkali, or organic compound, wash it immediately with water for 20 minutes. Remove clothing and jewelry. Do not try to neutralize it. Seek medical attention.

CHOLESTEROL PROFILE (BASIC)

Total cholesterol should be less than 200 mg/dl and should mainly consist of good cholesterol (HDL = high density lipoprotein) which is greater than 40 mg/dl and ideally more than 50 mg/dl. Bad cholesterol (LDL = low density lipoprotein) should be kept to less than 200 mg/dl, ideally less than 150 mg/dl.

CONVERSIONS

C = (5/9)(F - 32)
F = (9/5)(C) +32

1 in. = 2.54 cm
1 fl oz = 29.6 ml
1 qt = 0.946 L
1 g = 0.0035 oz
1 lb = 0.45 kg
1 cm = 0.394 in.
1 ml = 0.034 fl oz
1 L = 1.057 qt
1 oz = 28.38 g
1 kg = 2.2 lb
cal = "small" calories
kcal = kilocalories (Calories: 1 kcal = 1,000 cal)
Cal = "large" (dietary) calories (1 Cal = 1,000 cal)

Metric Measure of Length

1 meter (m) = 1000 mm or 100 cm
1 centimeter (cm) = 1 mm or 0.01 m
1 millimeter (mm) = 0.1 cm or 0.001 m

Metric Measure of Volume

1000 milliliters (ml) = 1 liter (L)
1 cubic centimeter (cc) = 1 milliliter (ml)

Metric Measures Of Weight

1,000,000 micrograms (mcg) = 1 gram (g)
1000 micrograms (mcg) = 1 milligram (mg)

1000 milligrams (mg) = 1 gram (g)
1000 grams (g) = 1 kilogram (kg)

Household Measure = Metric Measure
15 drops (gtt) = 1 milliliter (ml)
1 teaspoon (tsp) = 5 milliliters
1 tablespoon (Tbsp) = 15 milliliters
1 cup (c) = 180 milliliters
1 glass = 240 milliliters = 1 glass
22 pounds (lb) = 1 kilogram (kg) or 1000 grams (g)
1 inch = 2.5 cm
12 inches = 1 foot

Apothecary/Metric Equivalents

Metric Measure = Apothecary Measure
30 ml =1 fluid ounce (fl oz)
180 ml = 6 fluid ounces (fl oz)
240 ml = 8 fluid ounces (fl oz)
500 ml = 16 fluid ounces (fl oz) or 1 pint (pt)
1000 ml or 1 liter (L)=32 fluid ounces (fl oz) or 1 quart (qt)
60 or 65 milligrams (mg) = 1 grain (gr)
1 gram (g) = 15 grains (gr)
1000 grams (g) or 1 kilograms (kg) = 2.2 pounds (lb)

Multiply when a larger unit is converted to a smaller unit. Divide when converting a smaller unit to a larger unit.

CPT = Current Procedural Terminology

CPT designates any service rendered by a physician or qualified healthcare professional in an office, emergency department, hospital or nursing home.

CPT Modifiers are in front of the book with symbols and place of service.

1. Use the alpha index at back of book.

2. Use number tabs to find the procedure.

3. Remember the office and hospital services are placed in the front of the book. They are usually numbered from 99201 onward. They are like a chunk taken from the middle of the book and placed at the front.

If the procedure does not exist, report the service or procedure using the appropriate unlisted procedure or service code. Modifying or extenuating circumstances are added when necessary.

The medical record should adequately document any service or procedure.

CRUTCHES

A. Climbing Stairs

1. Use the good leg to step on the first stair.

2. Crutches and the bad leg should move together and sided by side when moving up a step.

B. Walking downstairs

1. Stand close to the edge of the step.

2. Adjust to the lower step by bending from the hips and knees to adjust to the height of the step.

3. Do not lean forward because it may cause a fall.

4. Carefully lower crutches and the affected leg to the lower step to resume balance.

5. If a handrail is available, use the two crutches on one hand and follow the steps above.

6. It is important to remember that the affected foot goes down first.

C. Sitting

1. Walk backward into the chair until it is against the backs of your legs (you will feel it).

2. Move both crutches to the hand on the affected leg and reach back for the chair with the hand on the side of the good leg.

3. Slowly lower yourself into the chair.

DEHYDRATION

Sx: Tachycardia, dry mouth, fatigue and low orthostatic blood pressure.

Tx: Replace salt and electrolytes (soup and Gatorade)

The average adult needs 2-3 liters of liquid a day. The patient may need intravenous fluid replacement if shock symptoms develop (malnutrition, acute blood loss, diarrhea, vomiting, sweating, fever which are all factors of cardiovascular volume depletion.

Common intravenous (IV) fluid replacements are isotonic solutions: normal saline (NS): contains 0.9% saline in 500-1000 cc.

D5NS: contains 50 gram/L of glucose and 0.9% saline
And Ringer's Lactate with calcium, potassium, salt and lactate.

DIABETES MELLITUS (DM)

IDDM: DM type 1 = insulin dependent

NIDDM: DM type 2 = needs to control diet and exercise and may take insulin or pills.

1. Ask the patient which medicine is taken, how many doses and at what times he takes them.

   Insulin: Fast acting (10 minutes to 4 hours): Humalog (Lispro)
   Regular (onset 1 hour, induration 6 hours)
   Slow Acting (onset 2 hrs, duration 24 hrs)
   Mixed 70/3 mixed 70% NPH and 30% regular)

2. Ask for the dates of the most recent: Ophthalmology exam, lab exam, foot exam, blood pressure check, (If more than 24 hours, the doctor may require a blood sugar (BS) check which should be labeled as "random" or "fasting". A finger stick for a glucose test should be done on the side of the finger because the tip is more sensitive and painful for the patient.

3. HYPOGLYCEMIA = not enough blood sugar (INSULIN REACTION) Patient signs: moody, confused, headache, perspiring, tremors, blood sugar is below 50, is able to have seizures or become unconscious.

   Tx: Immediately report this to an RN or physician and be prepared to feed him orange juice, honey, or candy if consciousness is present.

4. HYPERGLYCEMIA: Too much blood sugar (Diabetic Keto-Acidosis)

   Symptoms: weakness, confusion, nausea, vomiting, fruity (acetone) breath, dehydrated (dry mouth and poor urine output)

   Sugar>300
   pH>7.3
   serum bicarbonate<15 meq/L (See ABG's)

   Tx: Pt may need I.V. infusion and hospitalization. Refined sugar should be avoided and a consistent schedule should be used and adjusted for energy and activity.

EKG

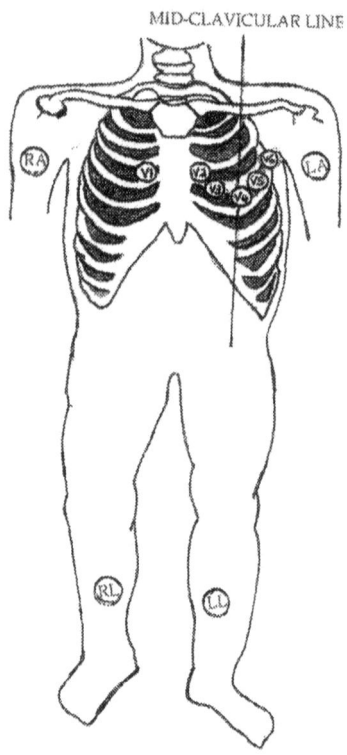

Patient needs to be bare from the waist upward with the exception of a gown that opens in the front. There must be direct access to skin on the lower legs. The two sets of electrodes and lead placement are usually labeled as follows:

1. Limb lead and electrode placement:

    LA = left arm
    RA = right arm
    LL = left leg
    RL = right leg

2. Chest (precordial) lead and electrode placement (V1 to V6):

   It may be necessary to shave the skin where electrodes are to be placed for good contact.

   Feel for the 4th ICS, feel for the first indentation below the collarbone and move your other fingers down three more spaces until four fingers are on the top intercostals spaces.

   V1 and V2 are placed on the 4th intercostal spaces of the right and left sternal margin.

   V4 goes on the mid-clavicular line and 5th ICS; it is often below the nipple.

   V3 is placed between V2 and V4.

   V5 is placed on the 5th ICS where the frontal axillary line begins.

   V6 is also on the 5th ICS along the middle of the axilla.

   Clamp all electrodes correctly. Have the patient securely placed with no limbs dangling. Ask him to be still and not to speak during the procedure.

   Enter patient's name and other data.

   Set speed at the 25 mm/sec.

   Turn on the machine by pressing run.

   Press the standard button for a pulse of 1 mV which will equal 10 small boxes on EKG paper. The rhythm strip is to be examined by the physician.

EKG lead codes

Lead	Code
I	.
II	..
III	...
aVR	-
aVL	- -
aVF	- - -
V1	-.
V2	-..
V3	-...
V4	-....
V5	-.....
V6	-......

FAINTING

If fainting has occurred, check ABCD (airway, breathing, circulation, disability), and position the victim on back with legs elevated 8 to 12 inches. If vomiting occurs or is anticipated, turn the victim on his side and loosen clothing surrounding the neck of the patient. Wipe the victim's forehead with a cool, wet cloth. If the victim has repeated attacks of unresponsiveness, loses consciousness while sitting or lying down, faints for no apparent reason, and/or does not quickly regain consciousness, seek medical attention. If the person is about to faint, prevent a hard fall if possible and lay the victim supine with legs elevated 8 to 12 inches. If vomiting occurs or is anticipated, turn the victim on the side and loosen clothing around the victim's neck. Wipe the forehead with a cool, wet cloth.

FEVER

Notify physician if temperature is 102 F or higher. Frequently check vital signs.

1. Take note of respiratory, skin or urinary infections or dehydration.

2. If the doctor wants CBC's and blood cultures done, do these first.

3. Although the illness must run its course before the temperature returns to normal, the temperature should be brought down to near 101 F for the patients comfort. (High fevers are often a natural defense against disease processes.)

Tx: use non-aspirin antipyretics prn (as needed) for comfort because aspirin has been implicated in Reye's syndrome in certain populations.

Comfort measures include resting in a quiet and dark room, eating a light diet, and consuming clear liquids if nausea and vomiting are present.

HCPCS ("Hick Picks")

This book is used for healthcare providers and medical suppliers to report professional services, procedures and supplies for reimbursement provided by physicians, therapists, home health, outpatient departments, and other caregivers. HCPCS is a catch-all-code classification. Chapters differ by service, and some are specifically for use by dentists, Blue Cross, outpatient prospective payment system hospitals and Medicaid.

The far left side boxed letter is a payment grouping that can be identified at the beginning of the book under APC status indicators and the 3 to 5 digit code is in the tabular list with service descriptions.

1. Look up the term for the service or procedure in the index in the front of the book. Use the table of contents for the type of procedure or device to narrow the code choices. Check the unlisted procedure guide for additional choices.

2. Use the tabular index to find all codes listed. (A single code, multiple codes, a cross-reference or an indication that the code has been deleted may be to the right of the terminology. All codes listed should be tentatively assigned.

3. Check for color bars, symbols, notes and references.

4. Review the appendices for definitions and other guidelines for coverage issues.

5. Determine if modifiers should be used.

6. Transfer or assign the code.

The back of the book contains modifiers, abbreviations, table of Drugs, and a National Coverage Determinations manual. HCPCS modifiers are also found on the inside front and back covers.

Do not code directly from the alphabetic index in the ICD-9-CM book.

HEAD INJURIES

1. Check ABCD (airway, breathing, circulation and disability) and check for possible spinal injury if the head is bleeding and a skull fracture is suspected, apply pressure to the outer edges of the intact bone.

2. If no fracture is suspected, apply pressure over the wound.

3. Immobilize the head and neck of the victim and do not remove any impaled objects.

4. If the head is not bleeding or you have controlled the bleeding enough, check for consciousness.

5. Raise the patient's head and shoulders if he or she is unconscious, there is no spinal injury and the patient is not in shock.

6. Seek medical attention.

Valeri S. Morimoto, BAE

HEARING

(complaints of ringing or hearing loss)

1. Identify patient and explain the procedure.

2. Test each ear with the headphones over one ear each time and then over both ears [right ear (AD)/left ear (AS)/both ears (AU)]

3. Begin with a low frequency and watch the patient for a sign of when the sound is heard. Plot this point on the graph.

4. Increase the frequency gradually until completed for that ear.

5. Give the graphic results of the test to the doctor for interpretation and findings.

If a patient can only hear decibels greater than 40, there is hearing loss.

1 below 20 dB = mild hearing loss
2 below 40 dB = moderate hearing loss
3 below 60 dB = severe hearing loss

Normal testing frequencies occur in Hertz (Hz) at 250/500/1000/2000/4000/8000

Normal hearing is between 0-20 dB

Decibels are units of loudness.

HEAT RELATED EMERGENCIES

HEAT EXHAUSTION

If a patient is exposed to excessive heat and has a normal temperature (skin is not hot), and normal mental status, it is heat exhaustion. Move the victim's legs 8 to 12 inches. Remove excess clothing and sponge the victim with cool water and fan. Give cold water or commercial electrolyte drink. Seek medical attention if no improvement within 30 minutes.

HEAT STROKE

1. If a patient has hot skin from excessive heat exposure, fever and altered mental status, it is heatstroke. Seek medical attention and move the victim to a cool place. Remove excess clothing. If humidity is high (greater than 75%) place ice packs on neck, armpits and groin.

   Stop cooling when status improves. Seek medical attention.

2. When humidity is less than 75% spray water on the victim's skin and vigorously fan the victim or cover the victim with a wet sheet or similar cloth. Keep the cloth wet and place ice packs on the neck, armpits and groin area. Stop cooling when mental status improves. Seek medical attention.

HEMORRHOIDS

Although hemorrhoids can bleed abruptly, they are not life threatening. They are a congested venous plexus of the rectal mucosa. External and Internal hemorrhoids are painful. Prolapsed hemorrhoids are protruding internal hemorrhoids that can be painful.

Tx: avoid prolonged standing or sitting.

Sitz bath for 20-30 minutes 2-3 times a day for pain decrease.

After bowel movements, creams or suppositories should be used that are either over the counter or prescription medicine.

ICD-9-CM = International Classification of Diseases 9th Revision Clinical Modification.

Descriptions of diseases, injuries, conditions and procedures.

1. Always use the alphabetic index and tabular list for accuracy.

   Use the alphabetic index in the front of the book to find the disease, injury or condition (dx or sx in the form of a noun, adjective or eponym). Do not code the symptoms that say "rule out, suspected, probable or questionable."

2. Interpret symbols, abbreviations, cross-references and brackets. NEC may follow some terms or subterms and means there is no code for the condition even if it is specific.

3. Use the longest code you can. They range from 3 to 5 digits. The longer the code, the more specific it is. (5 digits = fifth-digit subclassification codes, 4 digits = subcategory codes, 3 digits = category codes).

4. Identify reimbursement prompts and color coding for age, sex and Medicare as secondary payer in the official ICD-9-CM guidelines in back of book. Also refer to the AHA's Coding Clinic for ICD-9-CM for a guide in use of specific codes.

5. Transfer the code.

V and E codes in the back of the book are used to describe and support the regular code.

V codes = preventive measures (check ups, natural disasters and unforeseen circumstances)

E codes = motor vehicle accidents – injury category breakdown.

Appendices in the back of the book contain morphology of neoplasms, classification of drugs by AHFS list, classification of industrial accidents according to agency, and list of three-digit categories.

IMMUNIZATIONS

Recommended Schedule for Healthy Children and Infants

Age	Immunizations
Birth or 1 month	Hep B-1
2 months	DTaP or DTP, HIB, IPV, Hep B-2
4 months	DTaP or DTP, HIB, IPV
6 months	DTaP or DTP, HIB, Hep B-3
If a measles epidemic occurs, the first MMR can be given as young as follows.	
12-15 months	MMR, HIB
15-18 months	DTaP or DTP, OPV, VAR
4-6 years	DTaP or DTP, OPV
11-12 years	MMR
14-16 years	Td (repeat every 10 years) VAR (if susceptible, 2 doses 1 month apart)

ABBREVIATIONS

OPV: Oral polio vaccine

IPV: Inactivated polio vaccine

DTaP: Diptheria, tetanus, pertussis

DTP: Diptheria, tetanus, pertussis

Td: Full tetanus toxoid dose; half diphtheria dose

MMR: Measles, mumps, rubella

HiB: Haemophilus b conjugate vaccine

PnV: Pneumococcal vaccine

Hep B: Hepatitis B

VAR: Varicella vaccine

INJECTIONS (ID, IM, SQ, Z-track)

I.D. such as for a tuberculin TB test is given in a small 1.0 ml or 2.0 ml syringe. Cleanse the top of the Mantoux bottle with alcohol. Draw up 0.1 ml of air and inject air into the air portion of the bottle and turn the bottle upside down to withdraw the fluid just past the 0.1 mark. Flick air bubbles to the top and shoot air and 1-3 drops out of the bevel. Insert the needle at a 10-15 degree angle until the bevel is under the skin. Slowly inject the Mantoux fluid. A wheal should form.

SubQ, subcutaneous

(aspirate to see if you are in a blood vessel)

Use a small 2 cc or less syringe and a small 25-27 gauge needle with a length of ½ to 5/8 inches long. Insert the needle at a 45 degree angle all the way to the hub of the needle. Then slowly inject the medication and pull the needle out quickly.

Intramuscular, IM

(preferred sites are the deltoid, buttock, vastus lateralis)

Use a 2-5 cc syringe with a 20-23 gauge needle (usually 22g) that is ½ to 1 inch long. Insert the needle at a 90 degree angle all the way to the hub of the needle. Aspirate by pulling the plunger back and observe for blood in the syringe. If there is no blood, inject the fluid.

Z-track

(for IM injections with the preferred site in the buttocks)

This method is designed to prevent medication leakage from the needle tract. To accomplish this, pull the skin to one side and inject through the taut skin at a 90 degree angle. Remove the needle and release the pulled skin over the needle tract.

OTHER INTRAMUSCULAR SITES

Angle for IM (90 degrees), SQ (45 degrees) and ID (10-15 degrees) injections

INJECTIONS (ID, IM, SQ, Z-track)

Dorsogluteal Intramuscular (IM) site for injection

VENTROGLUTEAL INTRAMUSCULAR (IM) SITE

Intramuscular Sites

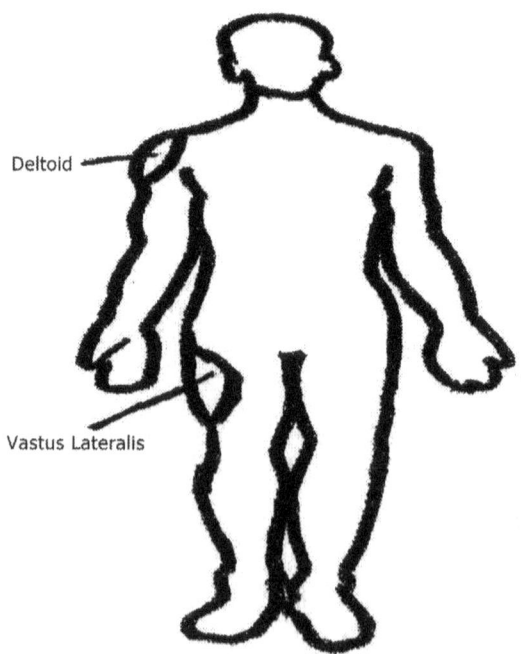

Injections (ID, IM, Z-track)

Dorsogluteal Intramuscular (IM) site for injection

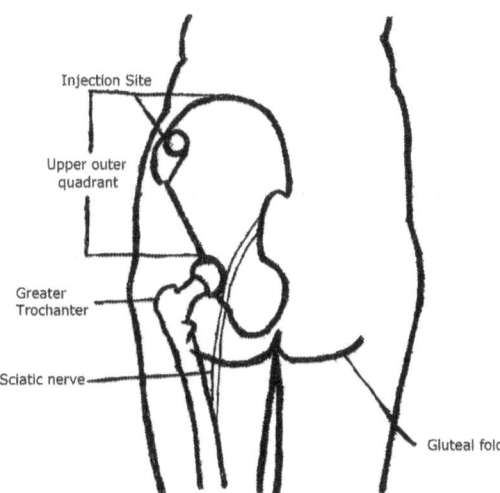

Ventrogluteal Intramuscular (IM) site

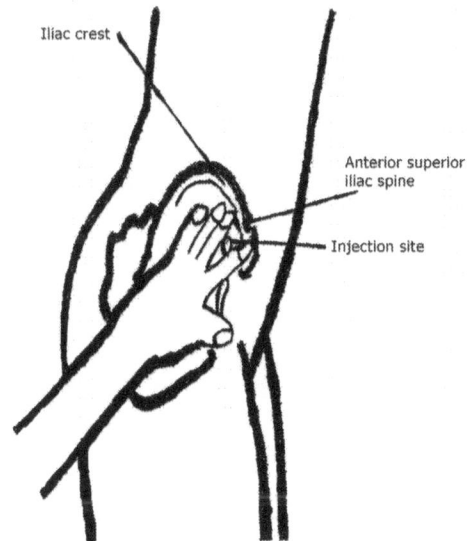

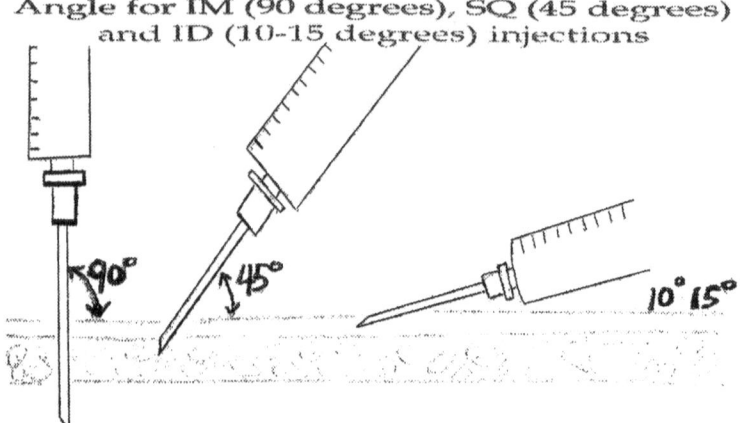

Angle for IM (90 degrees), SQ (45 degrees) and ID (10-15 degrees) injections

INSECT STINGS

If the stinger of a honeybee is imbedded in the patient's skin, scrape it off with a fingernail, credit card, or knife blade. Do not squeeze stinger.

If allergic to insect stings, seek medical attention immediately and keep the part lower than the heart.

If an epinephrine kit is available, follow directions before using. Monitor ABCs and treat accordingly.

If victim has no allergy to stings, watch for signs of allergic reaction. Wash the site with soap and water. Apply ice pack for 15-20 minutes. Relieve pain by giving aspirin (adult only) or acetaminophen. Relieve itching and swelling with topical steroid cream (hydrocortisone). Keep the stung part below the heart.

INTRAVENOUS INFUSION (ASSISTING)

1. Hang the bag of solution the doctor or registered nurse gives you on the I.V. stand loop at the top. Help to prime the solution if the Dr. or RN asks you to by eliminating air bubbles and running some of the fluid in the sink by releasing the roller stopper device. Close the stopper when there are no bubbles in the tubing.

2. Once the doctor or registered nurse has inserted the needle into the patients vein and connected the tubing to it, wait for the Dr. or RN to ask you to release the stopper. Then roll the stopper so it no longer clamps the tubing.

3. The infusion usually takes about an hour so check on the patient periodically as well as the amount of fluid in the bag.

4. When the bag starts to look about ¾ empty, remind the doctor that the bag is almost finished.

LETTERS, MEMOS & CARDS

TYPEWRITING

Elite and Pica (used by law offices) are the two main typewriter styles.

	ELITE	PICA
CENTER	51	42
Total Spaces	112	84
Pitch (acronym = characters per inch)	12	10

Letter Placement Table

Letter Classification	Side margins	Dateline Position
Short (up to ½ page)	2"	Line 18
Average (½ to ¾ page)	1½"	Line 16
Long (1 page or more)	1"	Line 14
2 page	1"	Line 14
Standard 6" line	1¼"	Line 16
Standard 6 ½" line	1"	Line 16

QS = 4 spaces between lines
TS = 3 spaces
DS = 2 spaces
SS = 1 space

Space twice if a sentence ends in ? or ! or .)

Use 2 or 0 spaces after a colon (To: person, or 8:30)

When centering letters on a page, count the spaces and divide by two and count back the divided number. If it is an odd number of letters, do not count back for a leftover stroke.

Space once after a comma (,) or semicolon (;).

When a deep letter head prevents the use of the indicated dateline position, place the date two spaces below the last line of the letterhead.

When letters contain special features or tables, adjust the dateline position upward on the letterhead.

If using a window envelope, the dateline position is on line 12. Some offices require the same line length and specific dateline position to be used for all letters, regardless of classification.

MODIFIED BLOCK

(line 16)

(51 spaces) Dateline

(4 spaces)
Name
Address
City, State, Zip Code
(2 spaces)
Salutation
(2 spaces)
Paragraphs: Modified Block Letter.
(2 spaces)
Complimentary Close
(4 spaces)

                        Name, title
                        Place
                        (2 spaces)
                        Initials of typewriter
                        (2 spaces)
                        Enclosure (if any)

This is a modified block letter format because the date, complimentary close and signature lines are positioned at the center point.

Use this format for personal letters and for those requiring indented paragraphs. Otherwise use the efficient, computer compatible block format.

BLOCK LETTER FORMAT
(also known as simplified block)

Dateline: 16
Left Margin: 18

DATELINE
(4 spaces)
NAME AND ADDRESS
SALUTATION
(2 spaces)
SUBJECT LINE
(2 spaces)
BODY
(2 spaces)
COMPLIMENTARY CLOSE
(4 spaces)
NAME
TITLE
(2 spaces)
INITIALS
(2 spaces)
ENCLOSURE

BLOCK LETTER (No Salutations such as Dear and To Whom It May Concern. There is also no complimentary close such as Sincerely. There is only a subject line and it can be sent to 100 people.)

The block format is useful when the name or title of the personal receiver of the letter is unknown and the company name must be used instead.

Sometimes the subject line is preceded and followed by a triple space. The simplified block letter format is computer compatible.

*Unless requested, block letters have no indentations for paragraphs. Instead a line is double-spaced between paragraphs.

Five spaces are used to indent paragraphs. However, do not indent a business letter. Only indent personal letters. The exception to not indenting a business letter is a modified block letter with indented paragraphs.

LONG LETTER FORMAT

Dateline: 14
Left Margin: 12

DATELINE
(2 spaces)
SPECIAL NOTATION (i.e. CERTIFIED MAIL)
(2 spaces)
COMPANY NAME
ATTENTION LINE (ATTN: person's name)
STREET ADDRESS
CITY, STATE, ZIP CODE
(2 spaces)
REFERENCE LINE (RE: …)
(2 spaces)
SALUTATION (Dear …)
(2 spaces)
SUBJECT LINE (If any)
(2 spaces)
BODY (flush left paragraphs separated by a double space)

NEXT PAGE (4 spaces from top edge of paper)
COMPANY NAME
PAGE #
DATE
(2 spaces)
PARAGRAPHS OF LETTER CONTINUED.
(2 spaces)
COMPLIMENTARY CLOSE (i.e. Sincerely)
(4 spaces)
SIGNATURE TITLE (Peron's name)
POSITION TITLE IN THE COMPANY
(2 spaces)
REFERENCE INITIALS (lower case)
(2 spaces)

ENCLOSURE NOTATION (Enclosure- if any)
(2 spaces)
COPY NOTATION (ie. c All employees)
(2 spaces)
POSTSCRIPT (i.e. See you in Hawaii)

**The second page of a letter begins 4 spaces from the top and requires:

Company Heading
Page 2
Date (DS)
Letter continuation.

Standard margins for all memos are LM = 18 & RM = 90)

STANDARD MEMO

Rules: Left margin=18, Right margin = 90, Dateline= 10, TO, FROM, DATE, SUBJECT = ALL CAPS)

Standard Memo

(10 spaces)
(13 spaces)To:
(double space)
(11 spaces)From:
(double space)
(11 spaces)Date:
(double space)
(8 spaces(Subject: (STANDARD MEMO)
(double space)
Paragraphs
(double space)
Initials

SIMPLIFIED MEMO

(10 spaces)
Dateline
(4 spaces)
To
(2 spaces)
Subject: SIMPLIFIED MEMO (ALL CAPITAL LETTERS)
(2 spaces)
Paragraphs (No indentations)
(4 spaces)
Name, title
Place
(2 spaces)
Initials
(2 spaces)
Enclosure

SMALL ENVELOPE

(1 space)
(2)MR. RETURN ADDRESS
2 ADDRESS STREET
HONOLULU, HI 99999-9999

1 inch left of center:

MR. FIRST LAST

(line 12 or 2 inches from the top) :

1 ADDRESS STREET
HONOLULU, HI 99999-9999

Folding And Inserting Letters Into Small Envelopes:

1. When letter is face up, fold the bottom up to 3/8 inch from the top.

2. Fold the sides into thirds from right side to left side.

3. Fold the left third up to ½ inch from the last crease.

4. Insert letter with the creased edge first.

LARGE ENVELOPE OR 10 INCH ENVELOPE

(1 space) |
(2 sp) MR. RETURN ADDRESS |
2 ADDRESS STREET (2 inches down)
HONOLULU, HI 9999-9999 |
|
MR. FIRST LAST
1 ADDRESS STREET
HONOLULU, HI 99999-9999

*The addresses are shown in the recommended style of the U.S. Postal Service.

Folding a letter into a large envelope:

1. Fold the bottom of the face of the page up to 1/3 from the top.

2. Fold the top third down 3/8 inch from the bottom crease.

3. Insert the letter with the bottom crease toward the bottom of the envelope so the flap will open up to the top of the face of the page.

MEDICATION FORMULAS

The West Nomogram method is considered the most accurate and is preferred for pediatric dosage for sick and underweight children. It can also be used for infants.

It is based on body surface area (height and weight.) The body surface area is expressed in square meters.

To calculate the BSA of a child, draw a straight line from the patient's height in inches or centimeters across the columns to the patient's weight in kilograms or pounds. The line will intersect on the BSA or SA column. The point of intersection gives the BSA average to be used in the formula for dosage.

BSA
Pediatric dose = $\dfrac{\text{basic surface area of child} \times \text{average adult dose}}{1.73 \text{ square meters}}$

FRIED'S RULE (12 months and under)
Pediatric dose = $\dfrac{\text{child's age in months} \times \text{average adult dose}}{150 \text{ months}}$

CLARK'S RULE
Pediatric dose = $\dfrac{\text{child's weight in pounds} \times \text{average adult dose}}{150 \text{ pounds}}$

YOUNG'S RULE (2 yrs to 12 yrs)
Pediatric dose = $\dfrac{\text{child's age in years} \times \text{average adult dose}}{\text{Child's age in years} + 12}$

Adult formulas:
D/A x Q = amount to give
(D= Desired, A= Available, Q= Quantity)

Or use the formula:

$$\frac{\text{Available strength}}{\text{Ordered strength}} = \frac{\text{available amount}}{\text{amount to give}}$$

MENTAL STATUS

Orientation to person, place and time is often documented as alert and oriented times the number or the three questions the patient answers correctly. "A&O X 1.2 or 3" depending on how many correct answers he or she gives to the questions.

VALIDATED BRIEF TEST

Ask the patient:

1. "What are three objects you remember?" [1 point]

2. "What year is it?" [1 point]

3. "What month is it?" [1 point]

4. "What day of the week is it?" [1 point]

5. "What were the three objects you named recently?"

TOTAL POINTS: 6

3 or more errors = high probability of dementia.
0 errors = unlikely cognitive impairment.

Callahan (2002) Med Care 40: 771-81

NOSEBLEED

If the nose was hit, suspect a fracture. Have the victim lean slightly forward to prevent blood from running down throat. Have the patient pinch nostrils together for 5 minutes. If the bleeding does not stop, ask the patient to gently blow nose and pinch nostrils together again for 5 minutes. If bleeding continues, apply ice and use a decongestant spray if available. If nosebleed continues, seek medical attention.

PAIN ASSESSMENT

Use the mnemonic PQRST

P: Provocative or palliative: "What causes the pain? What makes it feel better? What makes the pain worse?"

Q: Quality or quantity: "How does your pain feel look or sound, and how much pain is there?"

R: Region or radiation: "Where is your pain? Does your pain spread?"

S: Severity scale: "Does your pain interfere with activities?, How does your pain rate on a severity scale of 0 to 10, 0 being non-existent and ten being the worst?"

T: Timing: "When did your pain begin? How often does your pain occur? Is your pain sudden or gradual?"

PATIENT INTAKE

Have the patient fill out a face sheet for identification and insurance information. Most often, this is the HCFA-1500 (designed by the Health Care Financing Administration.) Claims processing at the insurance company requires the medical office to correctly and completely fill out the following items:

Name of the insured's insurance company
Name of insured
Insured's identification number
Address of insured
Telephone number of insured

The patient must sign a release of information to complete the form.

If the office requires a credit card to backup an insurance payment, have the patient sign and date the consent form.

Always greet the patient with a formal title of Mr., Mrs., or Ms. and their last name. Use first names after you have known them well enough or if they are younger than you.

Politely ask open ended questions such as: "How are you feeling today?" or "How may we assist you today?" and/or "What is the main reason you came in today?

Only write the chief complaint on the report form. You may put it in the patient's own words with quotations around it for legal matter or write your most accurate assessment. Remember, only the doctor can diagnose the patient.

Take the patient's blood pressure, pulse, respirations, and temperature. Ask if the patient has any known allergies (if none, write "NKA" for no known allergies.) Ask if the patient smokes or takes any medicine (Write down which ones if any). There may be an indication of "PMH" for past medical history. If the patient has had any surgeries, write it here. Then write the chief complaint for the visit. If there is any respiratory problem, take the patient's oxygen saturation and write in on the progress notes. If there is any mention of dysuria (painful or difficult urination),, do a UA dip and write the results such as color, pH, leukocyte, nitrite, keton, protein and blood results on the progress notes. Write your initials and military time the vitals signs were taken in the boxed area of the results. Write your name and title at the bottom of box of the chief complaint to indicate you took the patient's medical history.

PHYSICAL EXAM

Perform the following:

1. Multistix test on urine.

2. Blood draw with a lavender top (EDTA) tube for a specimen collection.

3. Ishihara (color vision) test.

4. Snellen vision test for far sightedness.

5. Vital signs

6. If patient is over 40 years old, perform an EKG.

7. If the patient is over 50 years old, perform or assist with a chest x-ray.

8. Anything else the physician requests.

POISON (SWALLOWED)

1. If conscious, identify the poison, quantity and time ingested. Call the poison control center or the medical source if it is a chemical or household product. Give milk or water.

2. If it is not a chemical, ask if you should induce vomiting.

3. If it is a chemical or household product, give syrup of ipecac (1 tbsp. for children less than 5 years old and 2 tbsp. for adults.) Give a glass of water with it.

4. After vomiting, give activated charcoal in premixed liquid form. Check ABC's (airway, breathing and circulation) and keep the patient on the left side to delay stomach emptying into small intestine.

5. If not instructed to induce vomiting, give activated charcoal in premixed liquid form if available. Check ABCs (airway, breathing & circulation) and continue to have the patient lying on his left side to delay stomach emptying into the small intestine.

6. If the patient is not conscious, check ABC's and treat accordingly. Lay the patient on his left side and seek medical attention.

PULSE

If a radial pulse cannot be felt on the thumb side of the wrist, listen for the apical pulse with your stethoscope on the midclavicular intercostals space on the patient's left side.

Other areas where a pulse can be felt are on the carotid artery (side of neck), femoral artery (upper thigh), brachial artery (antecubital fossa of forearm), popliteal artery (back of leg opposite of knee) and dorsalis pedis (upper foot), and tibialis posterior (lower outer portion of the tibia).

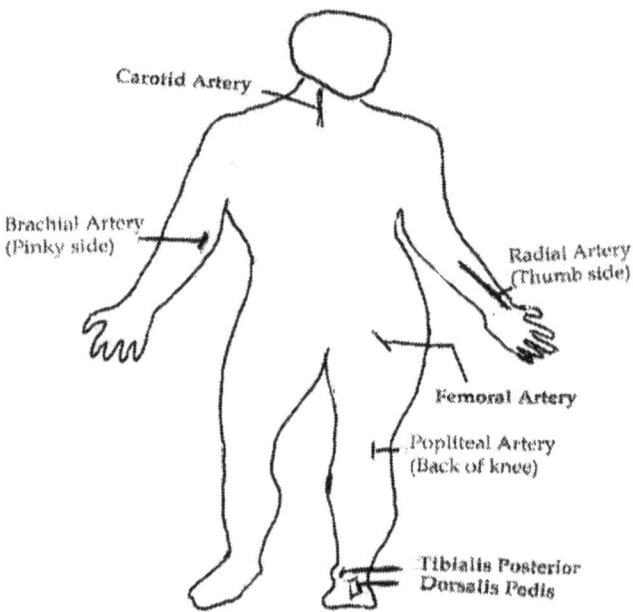

Take the pulse for a full minute to get an accurate reading.

RESPIRATIONS

1. Respirations per minute should be observed in a manner in which the patient does not realize it. An effective way to do this is to leave your fingers on the patient's wrist and watch the patient's torso on the stomach or chest for respiratory motion. One inhale and one exhale is one count.

2. If the patient needs supplemental oxygen, know where the oxygen tank is located and how to administer it when ordered.

3. If there is a pulse-oximetry machine in the clinic, know how to use it and realize a patient's position can affect its reading as in cases of orthopnea. Use the pulse oximetry device any time the patient complains of respiratory problems or if the respirations are not within normal range.

SEA URCHIN SPIKES

Patient's who stepped on sea urchin spikes may come in afraid of infection. Infection is rare. The medical assistant should obtain a plastic basin and fill it one inch high with very warm water and with about 3-10% white distilled vinegar for up to ½ hour. This will create a numbing effect to decrease pain on the sores. Have the patient lay on the surgery bed when the Dr. comes in for the procedure. Prepare a mayo stand with a beveled needle and sterile gauze. Be prepared to hand the doctor sterile gauze to absorb blood and to give him iodine soaked gauze for disinfection.

SEIZURES (CONVULSIONS)

1. Triage this patient or have an evaluation by a registered nurse or physician as soon as possible. Know the protocol for emergencies and location of the emergency cart, oxygen, EKG and IV's.

2. Monitor vital signs frequently and always have someone stay with the patient.

3. If there is a seizure (convulsion) do not restrain the patient. (you may help the patient to the floor).

4. Prevent injury by moving objects out of the way or by stopping a fall from the bed and by placing a mouthpiece in the victim's mouth to protect the airway and tongue.

5. Watch the patient for duration and type of convulsion.

    Simple Partial Seizure: local motor symptom.
    Complex Partial Seizure: consciousness impaired.
    Absence Seizure (Petit mal): Syncope (fainting) with a full tonic-clonic convulsion.

6. Notify the doctor immediately so he can arrange for hospitalization, medicine, etc.

7. When the seizure is over, position the patient in the Sims position (side-lying) and preferably on the left side to prevent vomiting due to the position of the stomach. The side lying position also helps to avoid aspiration and excessive salivation.

SHOCK

Shock is usually due to insufficient blood flow to vital organs which in turn creates the symptoms of low orthostatic blood pressure, altered mental status, fast heart and respiratory rate, low urine output, clammy and cyanotic skin.

Tx: maintain adequate oxygen and blood pressure, control pain, good urine output, and correct acid-base balance in ABG.

There are 6 types of shock:

1. Hypovolemic: burn, bleeding, severe fluid loss from pancreatitis, ascites and bowel obstructions.

2. Cardiogenic: congestive heart failure, arrhythmia and heart attack.

3. Obstructive: tension pneumothorax, pulmonary embolism.

4. Distributive: anaphylactic (acute allergic reaction)

5. Neurogenic (spinal cord injury)

6. Septic shock (infection)

SKIN CANCER

Check for A-B-C-D of Melanoma:

Asymmetry, border irregularity, color variation, diameter >6mm.

SPRAINS, STRAINS, CONTUSIONS & DISLOCATIONS

1. If the injury is located in a joint, check for a deformed appearance of the joint which will indicate a dislocation. If it is dislocated, check for circulation, sensation and movement. Stabilize the joint and seek medical attention.

2. If the injury is not deformed, it is a sprain, contusion caused by a blow to a muscle or a strain, apply cold such as crushed ice in a plastic bag for 20 minutes every 2 to 3 hours. Use RICE procedures of rest, ice compression and elevation. Compress the area with an elastic bandage to hold the cold package in place (not too tightly). Elevate the affected part above heart level.

3. If it is an injury from a blow to a muscle and there are uncontrolled muscle spasms such as cramps, have the patient drink mildly salted cold water. And apply an ice pack to the affected muscle. Gently stretch and/ or apply pressure. Cool compress for the first 24 hours to minimize swelling, pain and decrease bleeding or bruising. Heat or warm compress after 24 hours to decrease skin infection, increase circulation and speed healing.

SUTURES

Prepare the mayo stand with sterile gauze, clear tape, iodine, anesthetic, and a suture package. Move the surgery lamp so the spotlight is on the wound. Squeeze the anesthetic onto the physician's finger if he requests it.

TEMPERATURE CONVERSION

C = 5/9 (F − 32)

F = C (9/5) + 32

Document site temperature taken at
Orally (avg. 98.6) = po
Ear (avg. 98.6) = au
Rectally (avg. 99.6) = pr
Axillary (armpit avg. 97.6) = ax

THERMAL BURNS

(fire, hot objects or fluids)

1. If it is a severe burn and covers a large area, check ABCs (airway, breathing, circulation) and treat accordingly. Treat for shock and remove clothing and jewelry from the burned area. If the jewelry is stuck, cut it off. Do not pull it off. Apply a sterile dressing or clean cloth and elevate the burned arms or legs. Then seek medical attention.

2. If the severe burn is not a large area, apply a cold pack until the pain stops (10-40 minutes). Cover with nonstick, sterile dressing. Remove clothing and jewelry form burned area. Apply Bacitracin ointment. Check burn severity table as a guide about seeking medical attention.

3. If the burn is not severe, apply cold pack until the pain stops (10-40 minutes). Apply aloe vera or other moisturizer and check the burn severity table as a guide about seeking medical attention.

TUBERCULIN SKIN TESTING

1. Obtain the vaccination form and fill out the patient information.

2. Retrieve the TB testing fluid from the refrigerator, then a 10 ml syringe, an alcohol swab and gauze to wipe any excess after injection.

3. Escort the patient into the chair for injection.

4. Use any one of the forearms and select a site where the veins are not located.

5. Hold the skin taut beneath the injection site.

6. Perform an intradermal injection with the needle at a 10-15 degree angle.

7. Slowly inject the serum as it forms a wheal.

8. Fill out the vaccination form entering the site of injection, lot number, expiration date, date administered, your name and title.

9. When the patient returns in 48-72 hours, look for the induration (positive reaction of redness) and have the doctor examine it.

URINARY TRACT INFECTION (UTI)

Symptoms: Frequent urge to urinate with pressure and burning upon urination. Urine is red and odorous and patient has fever and upper back (flank) pain. Obtain some urine from the patient and do a multistix dip for analysis.

Positive signs of infection: red blood cells, white blood cells, bacteria, Nitrite, and a greater specific gravity than 1.03.

FYI (For Your Interest): Some patients have claimed that eating yogurt has relieved some UTI's due to an enzyme in it. Depending on the situation, cranberry juice has helped with some UTI's.

VAGINAL BLEEDING/MISSED PERIOD

1. Ask the patient for the last menstrual period (LMP), pap smear (LPS), or pregnancy. Ask what contraception the patient uses.

2. Gynecology history:

   Gravida = number of pregnancies
   Para = number of delivery
   Abortion = elective or therapeutic

3. Abnormal Paps:

   Class 1 (normal)
   Class 2 (inflammation
   ASCUS- Atypical Squamous Cells of Undetermined significance
   LGSIL- Low Grade Squamous Intraepithelial Lesion
   HGSIL-High Grade Squamous Intraepithelial Lesion
   CIN- Cervical intraepithelial neoplasia (suspicion for cancer)
   CIN I (low)
   CIN II (moderate)
   CIN III (high)
   Carcinoma in situ: presence of cancer

4. If the patient is bleeding, ask for the duration, amount of pads and tampons used daily and check vital signs. Obtain a urine specimen for a pregnancy test if needed. If a hemoglobin (Hemocue) machine is available ask the Dr. the pts hemoglobin should be checked.

5. Ask the patient to change into a gown and to remove the bottom half of clothing (pants or skirt) for a pelvic exam.

VENIPUNCTURE

1. Gather equipment: gloves, sterile gauze, alcohol swab, tourniquet, vacutainers and needles (20-25g) or syringes (10cc & 20cc) and butterfly needles. Select the blood tubes according to the proper colors for the tests desired.

2. The patient should have rested for 15 minutes prior to venipuncture because exercise and stress can cause high lactate dehydrogenase (LDH), AST, platelet count, and creatine kinase (CK) levels.

3. The patient should be in a lying or sitting position with the arm extended and slightly bent downward position to prevent backflow and fainting episodes.

4. Apply tourniquet 3-4 inches above site of injection Vigorous pumping of the hand should be avoided because it can cause hemolysis of hemoconcentration of particular analytes in the blood. Some gentle pumping is okay.

5. Palpate the vein you plan to use (the median cubital vein in the center and the cephalic vein on the thumb side are most common.) If you cannot feel one, apply the tourniquet tightly and put a warm compress on the site to cause the blood vessels to dilate for an easier draw.

6. Don gloves.

7. Clean the area with an alcohol swab and allow it to dry.

8. If using a syringe, open the syringe package and pull back on the plunger and push it all the way in to prevent excess air in the tube.

9. Hold the skin taut with your left thumb and index finger (or just your thumb). 1-2 inches below the puncture site to prevent the vein from rolling.

10. Hold the vacutainer or syringe tube with your thumb on top of the tube to insert the needle at a 15-30 degree angle with the bevel (slanted angle of the needle opening face up).

11. Insert the needle.

12. Release the tourniquet.

13. Advance the blood tubes into the vacutainer or slowly pull back from the syringe to draw blood from the patient.

14. Allow the tubes to fill to capacity.

15. Change tubes with the left hand if you are right handed, so you will not lose grip of the needle device.

    (Syringes and butterfly needles are suitable for fragile or thin veins and evacuated tubes are useful when larger amounts of blood are needed.)

    Remember the order of draw for an evacuated tube system (vacutainer):

    1. Yellow blood culture tubes or other tests for sterile specimens

    2. Blue stopper-coagulation tube

    3. Red top or red/gray or SST, gold or red-gray marbled stopper for nonadditive and gel separator.

    4. Green or light green stopper-Heparin tube with or without gel separator.

5. Lavender stopper- EDTA

6. Gray stopper-Oxalate/fluoride-antiglycolytic tube

SYRINGE ORDER OF DRAW

1. Yellow stopper for blood culture
2. Light blue stopper
3. Lavender stopper
4. Green stopper
5. Gray stopper
6. Red stopper

16. If you have not yet released the tourniquet, release it now. Do not leave the tourniquet on for more than 1-2 minutes because it can cause significantly high levels of cholesterol, iron, lipid, total protein, and AST levels. Prolonged tourniquet constriction may also cause hemoconcentration and possible hematoma (bruise) formation.

17. Remove the needle and apply sterile gauze.

18. Instruct the patient to put direct pressure on the site of the gauze for 3 to 5 minutes to prevent bruising. The patient may also be instructed to hold the puncture site above heart level. Flexing the elbow will also prevent clot bruising from venipuncture.

19. Check the site and apply a Band-aid if needed.

20. Invert tubes when required.

21. Label tubes immediately after the blood specimen has been drawn. Attach identification labels on tubes before leaving the side of the patient. Write the patient's name, identification number, date, time of collection, your initials & test requested.

WINGED INFUSION OR BUTTERFLY (double-pointed needle) METHOD

1. This draw is similar to the syringe or vacutainer Method and is the riskiest method for needle sticks.) However, the adapter or vacutainer is to be screwed on the needle of the tubing opposite of the one used for injection. Tape (two pieces) may be used to anchor the wings of butterfly to the site of injection. However, it is optional.

2. It may be necessary to use a red top nonadditive waste tube to clear the 0.5 ml of air in the butterfly tubing. If the tube is not filled because of this air, it will affect the additive to blood ratio.

3. If you are only using tubes for coagulation , use a "dummy" tube to collect blood first. This tube is to be discarded.

4. Hold each tube slightly down or horizontally to avoid transfer of additives from one tube to the next.

VISION

Far vision is generally tested as part of a complete physical exam and should be tested when there are any eye complaints such as infection, redness or pain.

1. The patient is to stand or sit 20 feet from the Snellen chart at eye level with usual prescription glasses or contacts on.

2. He should take the test with both eyes (OU), right eye (OD), and left eye (OS).

3. Have him or her read the third line and adjust the line read accordingly.

4. If the patient can read a line and has one character wrong, write a hyphen and the number wrong next to the ratio on the left side of the line read on the Snellen chart (i.e. 20/40-1 means one was wrong.)

5. Vision is compared to what a normal person can see at 20 feet. For example 20/40 means the patient can see what normal eyesight can see at 40 feet.

VITAL SIGN RANGES

TEMPERATURE

(The normal human temperature range is constant throughout life)

Fever Classification per oral readings:

Level	Fahrenheit (F)	Celsius/Centigrade (C)
Slight	99.6F-100.9F	37.6C-38.3C
Moderate	101.0F-101.9F	38.3C-38.8C
Severe	102.0F-104.0F	38.9C-40.0C
Dangerous	104.1F-105.8F	40.1C-41.0C
Fatal	106.0F-109.4F	41.1C-43.0C +

Body temperature ranges

Oral: 97.0F-99.0F
Rectal: 98.0F-100.0F
Axillary: 96.0F-98.0F

PULSE

PULSE PER MINUTE	AGE
80-180	NEWBORN
80-160	1 WEEK TO 1 MONTH
80-150	3 MONTHS TO 2 YEARS
75-110	2-10 YEARS
50-100	10 YEARS TO ADULT
60-80	ADULT
50-65	OLDER ADULT

BLOOD PRESSURE

AGE	BLOOD PRESSURE
NEONATE	Systolic 40-80 mmHg Diastolic 20-55 mmHg
NEWBORN TO 1 YEAR	65-91 50-56
2 TO 5 YEARS	90-95 55-56
6 TO 12 YEARS	96-107 57-66
13 TO 15 YEARS	109-114 63-67
16-18 YEARS	112-121 66-70
ADULT	90-140 60-90

Average Normal Blood pressure readings

Age Group	Average Blood Pressure (mmHg)
Newborn	50/25
6-9 years	95/65
10-15 years	100/65
16 to adult	118/76
Adult	120/80
Older Adult	138/86
Normal adult range	120/80

WEIGHT: (25-99 YEARS OLD)

MEN'S HEIGHT WITH 1 INCH SHOES	MEN WITH 5 POUNDS OF INDOOR CLOTHING	MEN + 5 #	MEN + 5 #
FEET/INCHES	SMALL FRAME	MEDIUM FRAME	LARGE FRAME
5' 2"	128-134	131-141	138-150
5' 3"	130-136	133-143	140-153
5' 4"	132-138	135-145	142-156
5' 5"	134-140	137-148	144-160
5' 6"	136-142	139-151	146-164
5' 7"	138-145	142-154	149-168
5' 8"	140-148	145-157	152-172
5' 9"	142-151	148-160	155-176
5' 10"	144-154	151-163	158-180
5' 11"	146-157	154-166	161-184
6' 0"	149-160	157-170	164-188
6' 1"	152-164	160-174	168-192
6' 2"	155-168	164-178	172-197
6' 3"	158-172	167-182	176-202
6' 4"	162-176	171-187	181-207

WOMEN'S HEIGHT WITH 1 INCH SHOES	WOMEN WITH 3 POUNDS OF INDOOR CLOTHING	WOMEN + 3 POUNDS	WOMEN + 3 POUNDS
FEET/INCHES	SMALL FRAME	MEDIUM FRAME	LARGE FRAME
4' 10"	102-111	109-121	118-131
4' 11"	103-113	111-123	120-134
5' 0"	104-115	113-126	122-137
5' 1"	106-118	115-129	125-140
5' 2"	108-121	118-132	128-143
5' 3"	111-124	121-135	131-147
5' 4"	114-127	124-138	134-151
5' 5"	117-130	127-141	137-155
5' 6"	120-133	130-144	140-159
5' 7"	123-136	133-147	143-163
5' 8"	126-139	136-150	146-167
5' 9"	129-142	139-153	149-170
5' 10"	132-145	142-156	152-173
5' 11"	135-148	145-159	155-176
6' 0"	138-151	148-162	158-179

1 Patient should remove all heavy items from his body.

2 Calibrate the scale by making it balance at zero.

3 Conversions:

Weight in pounds = Weight in kilograms 2.2

Kilograms X 2.2 (lbs)= Weight in pounds

22 pounds = 1 kilogram

0454 kg = 16 ounces (oz) = 1 lb
0028 kg = 1 oz = 28 g
1 kg = 1000 g = 2.2 lb = 35.2 oz
1 g = 0.03 oz

Lb	oz	lb	Oz
006	1	056	9
013	2	063	10
019	3	069	11
025	4	075	12
031	5	081	13
038	6	088	14
044	7	094	15
050	8	100	16

Example A: How many kg does a 100 # baby weigh?

100 X 0.454 = 45.5 kg

Or

100/2.2 = 45.5 kg

Example B: How many kilograms does a 6 pound 5 ounce baby weight?

Step 1: change 6 lbs into oz.

6# X 16 oz = 96 oz

Step 2: add 5 oz to 96 oz

5 + 96 = 101 oz

WOUNDS

1. Take vital signs and ask if patient has any allergies and when the last tetanus booster was.

2. Ask how, where and when the injury occurred. A separate medical form is sometimes needed for accidents, personal injury or work-related injuries.

3. Check if there is a possibility of a foreign body, other cuts or injuries.

4. Put pressure on the laceration site and open the dressing only when ordered by the doctor. Set up instruments for suturing. The smaller the suture number, the bigger the device is.

   Face and neck 5-0 or 6-0 sutures 5-7 days for removal
   Scalp and body 3-0 or 4-0 sutures 7-10 days for removal
   Hands and feet variable 10-14 days

   Treatment:

1. Minor surgical or closed wounds need a dressing on for 48 hours.

2. Change the dressing daily after a shower by removing the dressing and cleaning the wound with either hydrogen peroxide, a betadine swab or an alcohol swab to keep it clean and covered.

3. The wound should be allowed to dry before applying a small amount of Bacitracin or Neosporin and a new dressing. Do not use Vaseline or hydrocortisone.

4. If the dressing is sticking to the wound, moisten the dressing with saline or hydrogen peroxide to loosen the scab from the dressing.

5. Be observant for an increase in redness, swelling, pain, purulent drainage or fever which may indicate the wound is infected.

6. The physician should take care of wound debridements.

ABBREVIATIONS

1. AAA — abdominal aortic aneurysm
2. A&O — alert and oriented
3. AAS — acute abdominal series (X-rays)
4. AB, ab — abortion, antibodies, antibiotic
5. ABC — aspiration biopsy cytology
6. ABD — abdomen
7. ABG — arterial blood gas
8. ABO&Rh Factor — blood groups A, AB, B and O
9. ac — before meals
10. AC — air conduction
11. ACE — angiotensin 1 converting enzyme
12. Acc — accommodation
13. ACL — anterior cruciate ligament
14. ACTH — adrenocorticotropic hormone
15. AD — Alzheimer disease
16. AD, ad — right ear
17. ad lib — as much as needed ("ad libitum")
18. ADD — attention deficit disorder
19. ADH — antidiuretic hormone (vasopressin)
20. ADHD — attention deficit & hyperactivity disease
21. ADL — activities of daily living
22. AE — above the elbow
23. AF — atrial fibrillation
24. AFB — acid-fast bacillus (TB organism)
25. AFP — alpha fetal protein
26. AGE — acute gastro-enteritis
27. AGN — acute glomerulonephritis
28. AI — artificial insemination

29. AIDS	acquired immunodeficiency syndrome
30. AK	above the knee
31. ALB	Albumin
32. alk phos, ALP	alkaline phosphatase
33. ALL	acute lymphocytic leukemia
34. ALS	amyotrophic lateral sclerosis; also called Lou Gehrig disease
35. ALT	alanine aminotransferase (elevated in liver and heart disease); formerly SGPT
36. AMA	against medical advice
37. AMB	ambulatory
38. AML	acute myelogenous leukemia
39. ANA	antinuclear antibody
40. ANS	autonomic nervous system
41. ant	anterior
42. AODM	adult-onset diabetes mellitus
43. AP	anteroposteior
44. APTT	activated partial thromboplastin time
45. Aq	aqueous (in the form of liquid)
46. ARDS	acute respiratory distress syndrome
47. ARF	acute renal failure
48. ARMD, AMD	age-related macular degeneration
49. AS	aortic stenosis
50. as	left ear, aortic stenosis
51. asa	aspirin
52. ASD	atrial septal defect
53. ASHD	arteriosclerotic heart disease
54. ASO	anti-streptolysin O
55. AST	angiotensin sensitivity test; aspartate amino transferase (cardiac enzyme, formerly called SGOT)

56. Ast	astigmatism
57. AT	atraumatic
58. ATN	acute tubular necrosis
59. AU, au	both ears
60. AV	atrioventricular, arteriovenous
61. ax	axillary
62. Ba	barium
63. BaE	barium enema
64. baso	basophil (type of white blood cell)
65. BBB	bundle branch block
66. BC	bone conduction
67. BCC	basal cell carcinoma
68. BCP	birth control pill
69. BE	below the elbow. Barium enema
70. BEAM	brain electrical activity mapping
71. bid	twice a day
72. BK	below the knee
73. B/L	bilateral
74. BM	bowel movement, bone marrow
75. BP	blood pressure
76. BMR	basal metabolic rate
77. BNO	bladder neck obstruction
78. BP	blood pressure
79. BPH	benign prostates hyperplasia; benign prostatic hypertrophy
80. BRP	Bathroom privileges
81. BRBPR	bright red blood per rectum
82. BS	bowel sounds
83. BSE	breast self-examination
84. BSO	Bilateral-salpingo-oophorectomy
85. BTL	bilateral tubal ligation
86. BUN	blood urea nitrogen
87. BW	body weight
88. Bx, bx	biopsy
89. C&S	culture and sensitivity

90. C1, C2, and so on	first cervical vertebra, second cervical vertebra, and so on
91. CA	cancer; chronological age; cardiac arrest
92. Ca	calcium; cancer
93. CABG	coronary artery bypass graft
94. CAD	coronary artery disease
95. CAT	computerized axial tomography
96. cath	catheterization; catheter
97. CBC	complete blood count
98. CBG	capillary blood gas
99. CC	cardiac catheterization
100. CCU	coronary care unit
101. CDH	coronary heart disease
102. CEA	carcino-embryonic antigen carotid endarterectomy surgery
103. CF	cystic fibrosis
104. CHF	congestive heart failure
105. Chol	cholesterol
106. CK	creatine kinase (cardiac enzyme)
107. CLL	chronic lymphocytic leukemia
108. cm	centimeter
109. CML	chronic myelogenous leukemia
110. CMT	cervical motion tenderness
111. CMV	cytomegalovirus
112. CNS	central nervous system
113. C/O	complaining of
114. CO2	carbon dioxide
115. COPD	chronic obstructive pulmonary disease
116. CP	cerebral palsy, chest pain
117. CPD	cephalopelvic disproportion
118. CPK	creatine phosphokinase
119. CPR	cardiopulmonary resuscitation
120. CRF	chronic renal failure
121. C&S	culture and sensitivity
122. CS, C-section	cesarean section
123. CSF	cerebrospinal fluid

124. CT	computed tomography
125. CT scan,	CAT scan computed tomography scan
126. CTS	carpal tunnel syndrome
127. Cu	copper
128. CV	cardiovascular
129. CVA	cerebrovascular accident
130. CVS	chorionic villus sampling
131. CWP	Childbirth Without Pain
132. CXR	chest x-ray, chest radiograph
133. Cysto	cystoscopy
134. D	diopter (lens strength)
135. D&C	dilatation (dilation) and curettage
136. DC	discharge
137. DDD	degenerative disc disease
138. DDx	differential diagnosis
139. Decub	decubitus (ulcer); bedsore
140. Derm	dermatology
141. DI	diabetes insipidus; diagnostic imaging
142. Diff	differential count (white blood cells)
143. Dig	digoxin-heart medication
144. Dilantin level phenytoin,	seizure medication
145. DJD	degenerative joint disease
146. DKA	diabetic ketoacidosis
147. DM	diabetes mellitus
148. DNR	do not resuscitate
149. DOA	dead on arrival
150. DOE	dyspnea on exertion
151. DPT	diphtheria, pertussis, tetanus
152. DRE	digital rectal examination
153. DSAA	digital subtraction angiography
154. DTR	deep tendon reflexes
155. DUB	dysfunctional uterine bleeding
156. DVT	deep vein thrombosis
157. Dx	diagnosis

158. EBL	estimated blood loss
159. EBV	Epstein-Barr virus
160. ECG, EKG	electrocardiogram; echoencephalogram
161. ECT	electroconvulsive therapy
162. ED	erectile dysfunction; emergency department
163. EDC	estimate date of confinement
164. EDD	estimate date of delivery
165. EEG	electroencephalogram; electroencephalography
166. EGD	esophagogastroduodenoscopy
167. Em	emmetropia
168. EMG	electromyography
169. ENT	ears, nose and throat
170. eod	every other day
171. EOM	extraocular movement
172. Eos	eosinophil (type of white blood cell)
173. EPO	erythropoietin
174. ERCP	endoscopic retrograde cholangiopancreatography
175. ESR, sed rate	erythrocyte sedimentation rate; sedimentation rate
176. ESRD	end-stage renal disease
177. ESWL	extracorporeal shockwave lithotripsy
178. ETOH	ethanol, alcohol
179. EU	excretory urography; also called intravenous pyelography (IVP) or intravenous urography (IVU)
180. ex. Lap	exploratory laparotomy
181. ext	extremity, external
182. F/C	fever and chills
183. FB	foreign body
184. FBS	fasting blood sugar
185. Fe	ferritin/iron
186. FECG; FEKG	fetal electrocardiogram

187.	FHR	fetal heart rate
188.	FHx	family history
189.	FHT	fetal heart tone
190.	FROM	Full Range of Motion
191.	FS	frozen section
192.	FSH	follicle-stimulating hormone
193.	FTND	full-term normal delivery
194.	FT4-RIA	(free T4) Free Thyroxin
195.	FU	follow-up
196.	FUO	fever of unknown origin
197.	FVC	forced vital capacity
198.	Fx	fracture
199.	G	gravida (pregnant)
200.	GB	gallbladder
201.	GBS	gallbladder series
202.	GC	gonorrhea
203.	GER	gastroesophageal reflux
204.	GERD	gastroesophageal reflux disease
205.	GH	growth hormone
206.	GI	gastrointestinal
207.	Glu	glucose
208.	gm	gram
209.	GSW	gunshot wound
210.	GTT	glucose tolerance test
211.	gtts	drops
212.	GU	genitourinary
213.	GVHR	graft-versus-host reaction
214.	GYN	gynecology
215.	H-Flu	hemophilus influenza
216.	HA	headache
217.	HAV	hepatitis A virus
218.	Hb, Hgb	hemoglobin
219.	HBV	hepatitis B virus
220.	HCG	human chorionic gonadotropin
221.	HCT, Hct	hematocrit
222.	HCV	hepatitis C virus

223.	HD	hemodialysis; hip disarticulation; hearing distance
224.	HDL	high-density lipoprotein
225.	HDN	hemolytic disease of the newborn
226.	HDV	hepatitis D virus
227.	HEENT	head, eyes, ears, nose, throat
228.	HEV	hepatitis E virus
229.	HF	heart failure
230.	Hgb	hemoglobin
231.	Hgb-A1C	glycohemoglobin
232.	Hib	hemophilus influenza B
233.	HIV	human immunodeficiency virus
234.	HLA B27	human lymphocytic antigen
235.	HMD	hyaline membrane disease
236.	HNP	herniated nucleus pulposus (herniated disk)
237.	HP	hemipelvectomy
238.	HPI	history of the present illness
239.	HR	heart rate
240.	HRT	hormone replacement therapy
241.	hs	at bedtime
242.	HSG	hysterosalpingography
243.	HSM	hepatosplenomegaly
244.	HSV	herpes simplex virus
245.	HTLV-III	human lymphotropic virus, type III
246.	HTN	hypertension
247.	Hx	history
248.	I&D	incision and drainage
249.	IBS	irritable bowel syndrome
250.	ICP	intracranial pressure
251.	ICU	intensive care unit
252.	ID	intradermal
253.	IDDM	insulin-dependent diabetes Mellitus
254.	Igs, Ig (A,E,GM)	immunoglobulins (A,E,G,M)

255. I.M., IM	intramuscular; infectious mononucleosis
256. IMP	impression (synonymous with diagnosis)
257. IOL	intraocular lens
258. IOP	intraocular pressure
259. IPPB	intermittent positive-pressure breathing
260. IRDS	infant respiratory distress syndrome
261. IS	intercostals space
262. ITP	idiopathic thrombocytopenia purport
263. IUD	intrauterine device
264. IUGR	intrauterine growth rate; intrauterine growth retardation
265. IUP	intrauterine pregnancy
266. I.V, IV	intravenous
267. IVDA	intravenous drug user
268. IVF-ET	in vitro fertilization and embryo transfer
269. IVP	intravenous pyelography also called excretory urography (EU) or intravenous urography (IVU)
270. IVU	intravenous urography (IVU, also called excretory urography (EU) or intravenous pyelography (IVP)
271. JODM	juvenile-onset diabetes mellitus
272. JRA	juvenile rheumatoid arthritis
273. K	potassium (an electrolyte)
274. KD	knee disarticulation
275. KUB	kidney, ureter, bladder
276. L&D	labor and delivery
277. L1, L2, and so on	first lumbar vertebra, second lumbar vertebra, and so on
278. LAP	leukocyte alkaline phosphatase

279. LAT, lat	lateral
280. LBP	low back pain
281. LBW	low birth weight
282. LD	lactate dehydrogenase; lactic acid dehydrogenase (cardiac enzyme)
283. LDH	lactate dehydrogenase
284. LDL	low-density lipoprotein LH luteinizing hormone
285. LE	lupus erythematosis
286. LH	luteinizing hormone
287. LIH	left inguinal hernia
288. LLL	left lower lobe (lungs)
289. LLQ	left lower quadrant
290. LMP	last menstrual period
291. LOC	loss of consciousness
292. LP	lumbar puncture
293. LPS	Last Pap-smear
294. LS	lumbosacral
295. LSO	left salpingo-oophorectomy
296. Lt	left
297. LUQ	left upper quadrant
298. Lymphos	lymphocytes
299. MCH	mean corpuscular hemoglobin; mean cell hemoglobin (average amount of hemoglobin per cell)
300. MCHC	mean cell hemoglobin concentration (average concentration of hemoglobin in a single red cell)
301. MCV	Mean cell volume (average volume or size of a single red blood cell; high MCV=macrocytic cells; low MCV= microcytic cells)
302. MEG	magnetoencephalography
303. MG	myasthenia gravis
304. MI	myocardial infarction

305. Mix astig	mixed astigmatism
306. ml, ml	milliliters
307. MRA	magnetic resonance angiogram; magnetic resonance angiography
308. MRI	magnetic resonance imaging
309. MRI scan	magnetic resonance imaging scan
310. MRSA	Methicillin resistant Staph. aureus
311. MS	musculoskeletal; multiple sclerosis; mental status; mitral stenosis
312. MSG	monosodium glutamate
313. MSH	melanocyte-stimulating hormone
314. MVP	mitral valve prolapse
315. Myop	myopia
316. N/V/D/C	nausea/vomiting/diarrhea/constipation
317. Na+	sodium (an electrolyte) NB newborn
318. NAD	no active disease/no acute distress
319. NCV	nerve conduction velocity
320. NG	nasogastric
321. NGU	non-gonococcal urethritis
322. NIDDM	non-insulin-dependent diabetes mellitus
323. NIHL	noise-induced hearing loss
324. NKA	no known allergies
325. NKDA	no known drug allergy
326. NPO	nothing by mouth
327. NMTs	nebulized mist hearing loss
328. NS	nervous system, normal saline
329. NPH	neutral protamine Hagedorn (insulin)
330. npo	nothing by mouth

331. NSAIDs	nonsteroidal anti-inflammatory drugs
332. NSVD	normal spontaneous vaginal delivery
333. NT	nontender
334. O&P	ova & parasite
335. O2	oxygen
336. OB	obstetrics, occult blood
337. OCPs	oral contraceptive pills
338. OD	right eye
339. OD	Doctor of Optometry
340. OM	otitis media
341. OOB	out of bed
342. OR	operating room
343. ORTH, ortho	orthopedics
344. OS	left eye
345. OU	both eyes together
346. P	phosphorous; pulse; para (number of babies born)
347. PA	posteroanterior; pernicious anemia
348. PAC	premature atrial contraction
349. Pap	Papanicolaou smear
350. Para 1,2,3	unipara, bipara, tripara (number of viable births)
351. PAT	paroxysmal atrial tachycardia
352. Pc, pp	after meals (postprandial)
353. PCL	posterior cruciate ligament
354. PCNL	percutaneous nephrolithotomy
355. PCO2	partial pressure of carbon dioxide
356. PCP	Pneumocystis carinii pneumonia
357. PCV	packed cell volume
358. PE tube	pressure-equalizing tube (placed in the eardrum)
359. PERRLA	pupils equal, round and reactive to light and accommodation
360. PET	positron emission tomography

A Handbook for Medical Assistants and Medical Secretaries

361. PFT	pulmonary function tests
362. PGH	pituitary growth hormone
363. pH	symbol for degree of acidity of alkalinity
364. PID	pelvic inflammatory disease
365. Plt	platelet count
366. PMH	past medical history
367. PMP	previous menstrual period
368. PMS	premenstrual syndrome
369. PND	paroxysmal nocturnal dyspnea
370. po	by mouth (per os)
371. POD	post-operative day
372. PO2	partial pressure of oxygen
373. Poly, PMN, PMNL	polymorphonuclear leukocyte
374. Post	posterior
375. PPD	purified protein derivative
376. PRL	prolactin
377. Pr	by rectum
378. prn	as required
379. PRBC	packed red blood cells
380. Prl	prolactin
381. prn	as needed ("pro re nata")
382. pt	patient
383. PSA	prostate-specific antigen
384. PT	prothrombin time, physical therapy
385. PTCA	percutaneous transluminal coronary angioplasty
386. PTH	parathyroid hormone; also called parathormone
387. PTT	partial thromboplastin time
388. PUD	peptic ulcer disease
389. PVC	premature ventricular contraction
390. q	every ("quaque")
391. q2h	every 2 hours
392. qam, qm	every morning

393. qd	every day
394. qh	every hour
395. qid	four times a day ("quarter in die")
396. qod	every other day
397. qpm, qn	every night
398. R/O	rule out
399. RA	rheumatoid arthritis, right atrium
400. RAI	radioactive iodine
401. RAIU	radioactive iodine uptake
402. RBC, rbc:	red blood cell (erythrocyte), red blood count.
403. RD	respiratory distress
404. RDA	recommended daily allowance
405. RDS	respiratory distress syndrome RF rheumatoid factor
406. Retic.	Reticulocyte count
407. RF	rheumatoid factor
408. RK	radial keratotomy
409. RLL	right lower lobe (lungs)
410. RLQ	right lower quadrant
411. ROM	range of motion
412. RP	retrograde pyelography
413. RSO	right salpingo-oophorectomy
414. rt	right
415. RTC	return to clinic
416. RUL	right upper lobe (lungs)
417. RUQ	right upper quadrant
418. RV	residual volume; right ventricle
419. Rx	treatment, prescription
420. S	without ("sine")
421. sAB	spontaneous abortion
422. SA	sinoatrial
423. SaO2	arterial oxygen saturation
424. SBE	self breast exam, heart infection
425. SBFT	small bowel follow through
426. SD	shoulder disarticulation
427. Segs	segmented neutrophil

428. SGGT	serum gamma-glutamyl Transpeptidase
429. SGOT	serum glutamic-oxaloacetictransaminase
430. SGPT	serum glutamic-pyruvic transaminase
431. SI	suicidal ideation
432. SICS	small incision cataract surgery
433. SIDS	sudden infant death
434. sig	write on label ("signa")
435. SL	sublingual (underneath tongue)
436. SLE	systemic lupus erythematosus
437. SNS	sympathetic nervous system
438. SOB	shortness of breath
439. Sp.gr.	specific gravity
440. SPECT	single photon emission computed tomography
441. SQ/SC	subcutaneous
442. S/S	signs and symptoms
443. ST	esotropia
444. stat	immediately
445. STD	sexually transmitted disease
446. Sub-Q, subQ	subcutaneous (injection)
447. Sx	symptoms
448. Sz	seizure, convulsion, epilepsy
449. T&A	tonsillectomy and adenoidectomy
450. T3	triiodothyronine (thyroid hormone)
451. T4	thyroxine (thyroid hormone)
452. TAH	total abdominal hysterectomy
453. TBG	thyroid-binding globulin
454. TB	tuberculosis
455. TCB	to come back
456. Tbsp.	tablespoon (15cc)
457. Td	tetanus-diptheria toxoid
458. TFT	thyroid function test

459.	THA	total hip arthroplasty
460.	THR	total hip replacement
461.	TIA	transient ischemic attack
462.	TIBC	total iron binding capacity
463.	tid	three times a day
464.	TKA	total knee arthroplasy
465.	TKR	total knee replacement
466.	TM	tympanic membrane, ear drum
467.	TMJ	temporal mandibular joint
468.	TOPV	trivalent oral polio vaccine
469.	TPR	temperature, pulse, and respiration
470.	TSE	testicular self-examination
471.	TSH	thyroid-stimulating hormone
472.	TURP	transurethral resection of the prostate (for prostatectomy)
473.	TVH	total vaginal hysterectomy
474.	Tw	twice a week
475.	Tx	treatment, transplant
476.	U&L, U/L	upper and lower
477.	UA	urinalysis
478.	UC	uterine contractions
479.	UGI	upper gastrintestinal
480.	Ung	ointment
481.	URI	upper respiratory infection
482.	US	ultrasound
483.	UTI	urinary tract infection
484.	VA	visual acuity
485.	VC	vital capacity
486.	VCUG	voiding cystourethrography
487.	VD	venereal disease
488.	VDRL	venereal disease research lab
489.	VF	visual field
490.	VSD	ventricular septal defect
491.	VSS	vital signs stable
492.	VT	ventricular tachycardia
493.	Vx	vaccination

494. WBC, wbc	white blood cell, white blood count
495. WD	well-developed
496. WF	white female
497. WI	walk in, without appointment
498. WM	white male
499. WN	well-nourished
500. WNL	within normal limits
501. w/u	work up, under investigation
502. XP, XDP	xeroderma pigmentosum
503. XRT	external radiation treatment
504. XT	exotropia
505. ZE	Zollinger-Ellison syndrome

GLOSSARY

ABA number: Bank identifying code number on the top right corner of a check
Abandonment: Discontinuation of patient treatment without providing coverage or sufficient notice of withdrawal.
Accession: Numbers recorded and assigned to each new patient name.
Accounting: Reporting method of financial results of a business.
Accounts receivable: Money due to the physician/ medical Practice.
Accreditation: When a school voluntarily completes a thorough self-study and an accrediting association then visits to verify the self-study statements.
Acquired immune deficiency syndrome (AIDS): Series of infections resulting from infection by the human immunodeficiency virus (HIV) which eventually causes the immune system to break down.
Active: Medical files of patients currently being seen by the physician (covering from 1-5 years depending on office policy).
Active voice: When the subject of the sentence performs the action.
Acuity: Sharpness or clearness of vision.
Acute condition: Condition with sudden onset, severe symptoms and short course.
Addiction: Acquired psychological and physical dependence on a drug.
Administrative: Business functions of a physician's office.
Aerobes: Microorganisms requiring oxygen to live.
Affect: Emotional state of a patient.
Age analysis: A process of evaluating accounts receivable by age.
Agent: Person acting on behalf of another person.
Agglutination: Process of clumping.

Aggressive: Violent style of convincing one to agree.
Agranulocyte: white blood cell with clear cytoplasm.
Alleged: Declaring without proof.
Allergen: substance triggering an allergic reaction.
Alphabetic: filing pertaining to letters of the alphabet.
Alveoli: air sacs in lungs for gas exchange between alveolar air and pulmonary capillary blood.
Ambulatory care: health care for those not hospitalized.
Ambulatory surgery: surgery without an overnight stay.
American Association of Medical Assistants (AAMA): Professional association for medical assistants overseeing program accreditation.
American Medical Association (AMA): Professional association for physicians to maintain directories of all qualified physicians, evaluates drugs and advises congressional and state legislatures for proposed health care laws and publishes scientific journals.
American Medical Association (AMT): Professional association overseeing registration of medical technologists.
Amplify: to increase in power or sound.
Amplitude: degree of voltage up or down when recording the electrical output of the heart.
Anaerobes: microorganisms not requiring oxygen to live.
Anaphylactic shock: life-threatening reaction to foods, drugs and insect bites that cause respiratory distress, edema, rash, convulsions and eventually unconsciousness and death if emergency treatment is not performed.
Anemia: decrease in circulating RBCs.
Anesthesia: loss of sensation partial or complete.
Aneurysm: When a wall of an artery weakens or out-pouches.
Angiography: X-ray view of the heart and blood vessels after injection of a radiopaque material in the blood vessels.
Anorexia: loss of appetite for food.
Antecubital fossa/space: inside bend of the elbow.
Anthrax: A deadly infectious disease contracted by humans through infected animal hair, hides or waste. It is deadly and infectious.

Anthropometric: human measurements such as height and weight.
Anthropometry: Science of measuring human body size of parts, height and weight.
Antibodies: Proteins defending infection of the body.
Anticoagulant: (EDTA and heparin) Substance to prevent blood form clotting.
Antigen: Foreign substance helping to produce antibodies.
Antipyretic: Fever reducing substance.
Apothecary system: System of weights and measures based on the basic units of grain, gram and dram.
Appellant: One who appeals a court decision by going to a higher court?
Archives: records stored for legal purposes that are no longer needed. (i.e. death records, inactive patients).
Aromatic: natural or pleasant odor.
Arraignment: When one is called before a court to answer a charge.
Arrhythmia: Irregular heart rate or pulse.
Artifact (s): Deflections in an EKG reading from other than from the heart being irregular and erratic.
Artificial insemination: Semen placed in the vagina without sexual intercourse.
Artificial insemination donor (AID): Donor of semen other than the husband or partner.
Artificial insemination husband (AIH): Husband's semen is used for pregnancy.
Aseptic: No germs.
Asphyxia: Inability of breathing (suffocation)
Aspirated: Drawn in or out by vacuum.
Assertive: A positive manner of declaring.
Assessment: Evaluation
Assignment of benefits: Written authorization of the patient for the insurance company to pay the physician directly for billed charges.
Asymptomatic: Without symptoms
Attitude: Mental disposition
Atypical: Not ordinary

Audit: Examination of records.
Aural: Pertaining to hearing or the ear.
Auscultatory gap: An abnormal and complete loss of sound in phase II of the Korotkoff sounds which later recurs when taking a blood pressure.
Autopsy: Examination of a person's organs and tissues to determine the cause of death.
Axilla: armpit
Bacteria: Microorganism able to cause disease.
Bactericidal: able to destroy bacteria that causes disease.
Baseline: Isoelectric line (flat on the electrocardiogram)
Batch transactions: In medical computes, one day's business in a set of transactions for a clinic.
Benefit period: When payments for Medicare inpatient hospital benefits are available.
Benign: Not cancerous.
Biopsy: Tissue sample for examination for cancer cells.
Bipolar disorder: Mental disorder of manic-depression.
Blind ad: When only a post office box is advertised for a position in a classified ad.
Block: Letter writing style of a flush left tendency.
Blood culture: Blood specimen upon media to promote growth for diagnosis of specific diseases.
Blood relative: birth lineage relation.
Blood stasis: Stoppage of blood flow.
Bloodborne pathogens: Microorganisms the produce disease and are transmitted through blood and body fluids containing blood.
Body mechanics: Techniques of standing and lifting objects to avoid fatigue and injury.
Bookkeeping: Maintaining accounts of the medical office.
Borderline hypertension: Gradually elevated blood pressure over a period of time until it borders the edge of high blood pressure.
Bradycardic: Relating to an abnormally slow heart rate of less than 60 beats per minute.

Breach of contract: A failure to comply with all terms in a valid contract.
Broad-spectrum: Drug ability to be effective against a wide range of microorganisms.
Buffy coat: A white coat composed of WBCs and platelets separating the packed RBCs and plasma after a whole blood specimen has been centrifuged.
Bulimia: Eating disorder of recurrent binge eating and then a purging of food with laxatives and vomiting.
Bureau of Narcotics and Dangerous Drugs (BNDD): Federal government used to enforce drug control.
Cadaver: a deceased body or a corpse.
Caduceus: symbol of healing composed of a staff with two snakes coiled around it, now a recognized symbol for healing.
Canceled checks: deposited checks already processed by the bank.
Capillaries: Minute blood vessels which connect arterioles and venules.
Cardiac cycle: Time beginning from one heart beat to the next beat to include the systole (contraction) and diastole (relaxation). One heart beat arbitrarily designed as P,Q,R, S, and T, consisting of contraction and relaxation of both atria and ventricles making one pulse.
Cardiac rate: Number of contractions or beats per minute; pulse rate.
Carrier(s): One who is capable of transmitting a disease and is unaware he or she has it.
Case law: Law established in prior cases.
Catheterization: Inserting a sterile tube into the bladder for urine withdraw or into a vein for an infusion procedure.
Caustic: Capable of eating away or burning tissue.
Censure: To criticize, condemn, or find fault with.
Centigrade or Celsius: Temperature scale in which 0C is the freezing point of water and 100C is the boiling point of water at sea level.
Centrifuge: A machine for separating blood into its liquid and solid components.

Cerebrovascular accident: Hemorrhage in the brain which may result in loss of speech or paralysis.
Certification: Issuance of a certificate by an official body indicating evaluation and a meeting of certain standards.
Certified: declared, confirmed or verified.
Certified medical assistant (CMA): A healthcare professional who is multi-skilled and assists providers in an allied health care setting and successfully completes a CMA certification examination validating his or her credentials.
Channel: A pathway for one signal is a channel.
Chemotherapy: Treating or controlling infections and diseases with the use of chemicals including drugs; often used to treat cancer by killing the cells.
Cholera: An acute infection pertaining to the small bowel which causes severe diarrhea.
Chronological: An arrangement of events in an order.
Circumcised: Foreskin surgically removed from the surrounding of the glans penis.
Citation: To quote from an authority.
Civil case: Court action not involving a crime and between private parties, corporations, or government bodies.
Claim: Documented request for reimbursement of an eligible expense under an insurance plan.
Claustrophobia: Fear of narrow or closed-in spaces.
Clinical: Pertaining to the medical treatment of patients.
Closed: Medical files of patients who indicate they will not be patients or who have died. For legal reasons, these files are kept in storage.
Code of ethics: Statement of guidelines for moral behavior.
Coding: Transferring narrative description of diseases and procedures into numbers. A coinsurance plan will pay a percentage of eligible benefits after a deductible has been paid.
Coinsurance: A cost-sharing provision requires the insured to pay some of the cost of covered services.
Collating: To gather and group materials by category.
Colleague(s): a fellow member in a profession.
Command: An order made on a computer for a function to activate.

Colostomy: A surgical opening into the large bowel for the removal of waste (feces).
Competent: Ability to manage one's own affairs.
Complex: Multiple deflections or waves occurring in a group.
Condescending: Authoritative implication.
Confidentiality: Keeping private information from being disclosed to third parties.
Consent: Permission or approval Consent, implied; inference by inaction, silence or signs that consent is granted.
Consent, infomed: Knowledgable consent by a patient based on the understanding of potential risks and benefits provided by the physician prior to surgery.
Consideration: Benefit or inducement that compels a person to enter into a contract.
Contagious: Transmittable diseases able from one person to another.
Continuing education units: (CEUs)
CPT code: Current Procedural Terminology listing describing terms and identifying codes for reporting medical services and procedures of physicians.
CPU: Central Processing Unit; Arithmetic operations and data processing part of the computer system.
Continuing education units (CEUs): Credit for additional education beyond certification to remain current in one's field or for recertification.
Credit: When added to an account to reduce an amount owed.
Criminal case: Court action from the state against persons or groups of people accused of committing a crime, resulting in a fine or imprisonment if found guilty.
Criteria: A standard to compare for a decision.
Crossover claim: Medi/Medi. When a patient qualifies for both Medicare and Medicaid.
Croup: Acute viral infection in children of the upper and lower respiratory tract resulting in difficult, noisy breathing.
CRT: Cathode Ray Tube; a tube of electronics; front of the screen of a 911 terminal.

Cryosurgery: Use freezing temperatures to probe or destroy abnormal cells.
Cultures(s): The regenerating of microorganisms or of living tissue cells in a special media conducive to their growth and/or the process by which organisms are grown on media and identified.
Culturette: Self-contained culture packet system that adapts to most office specimen collections from the throat, nose, eye, ear, rectum, wound and urogential sites. It has a disposable, sterile plastic tube containing a cotton-tipped applicator swab and a sealed ampule of Stuart's holding medium.
Cumulative: Exposure of a substance adds to the effect of all previous exposures.
Cumulative action: The action occurring in the body when a drug is allowed to stay or accumulate in the body.
Currency: Legal paper money.
Cursor: small, bright rectangle that indicates where the next entry will be accepted on the screen.
Cyanosis: Transmittable diseases from one person to another.
Cytology: Science dealing with formation, structure and function of cells.
Damages: Compensation for an injury or loss.
Data: Information, statistics or figures.
Debit(s): money owed; a charge.
Deductible: Percentage of charges a patient must pay for each calendar year before the plan begins to pay benefits.
Default: An entry a computer assumes that the operator can override.
Defendant: The accused in a court of law.
Defensive behavior: Reaction to a perceived threat either conscious or unconscious.
Deflection: Deviation up or down from the isoelectric line or from zero.
Dehydration: Body water loss that can become life-threatening if not corrected.
Delete: To erase.

Demographic: Data pertaining to descriptive information such as age, gender, ethnic background and education.
Depolarization, atrial: Electrical activity discharge in the upper heart chambers.
Depolarization, ventricular: Electrical activity discharge in the lower chambers.
Depolarized (depolarization): Electrical activity discharge that precedes contraction.
Deposit: Placing money into a bank account.
Deposition: Written statement of oral testimony made before a public officer of the court for use in a lawsuit.
Diagnose: To determine the nature and cause of a pathological condition.
Diagnosis code: An established standardized number to identify defined diagnoses for physicians.
Diagnostic: An evaluation, series of tests or a test to determine the extent of an illness or disease.
Diagnostic Related Groups (DRGs): Designations for identifying reimbursement per condition in a hospital used for Medicare patients.
Diaphragm: Musculofibrous partition that separates the thoracic and abdominal cavities.
Diastole: Period in the cardiac cycle when the heart is relaxed and the heart cavities are being refilled with blood.
Diathermy: Use of heat-inducing wave-lengths for muscle relaxation and therapy.
Differential diagnosis: Distinction between alternative diagnoses being two or more.
Digestion: Process of breaking down food mechanically and chemically in the alimentary canal.
Dilute: Weakening the strength of a substance by the addition of something else.
Disbursement: Payment of money or funds.
Discriminatory: To make someone separate or act with prejudice against a group.
Disk: Data and software medium for storage.
Draft: A writing prior to a final revision.

Drug tolerance: A decrease in a drug's effectiveness after continued use of the drug.
Duty: Responsibility or obligation.
Dyspnea: labored or difficult breathing.
Dysuria: Pain upon urination.
Editing: Restatement or rearranging of a word or group of words in a document.
Electrocardiogram: A recording of voltage or electrical activity with respect to time
Electrode: Sensor to detect electrical charges.
Electrolyte(s): 1.Ionized salts in blood such as Na, K and Cl. 2. Material applied to the skin enhancing contact between skin and sensor.
Emancipated minor: One under age 18 who is free of parental care and financially responsible for herself or himself.
Embezzlement: Breaching trust by taking money.
Empathy: To imagine how another person is feeling.
Emphysema: abnormal pulmonary condition from loss of lung elasticity that results in overinflation of the lungs and difficulty exhaling. Also know as "barrel chest."
Endocardium: Endothelial membrane that lines the chambers of the heart.
Erythemia: Skin redness.
Erythrocyte: An RBC or red blood cell.
Escherichia coli (E. coli): Bacillus in the colon or intestine that can cause infections when it is present in the urinary tract.
Ethics: Guidelines for moral behavior.
Evaluation: Judgement or assessment.
Expert witness: A medical practitioner who gives testimony about in court on a subject he or she has special knowledge from experience, training or education in and usually for a fee.
Expulsion: An act of forcing out.
Externship: On-the-job training through a school connection while not being paid.
Extracurricular: Activities performed along side and separate from academic requirements.

Exudates: Accumulation of serum, pus or fluid in a cavity or tissue which may become hard and crusty.
Facsimile (fax): A document of print and/or graphic information that ahs been electronically transmitted.
Fahrenheit: Temperature scale of measurement where the boiling point of water is 212F and the freezing point of water is 32F at sea level.
Family Chain: A group of records capable of designating patients as HEAD OF HOUSE or FAMILY MEMBER when they are linked together.
Feces: stool
Fee schedule: How much a specific insurance will pay for each procedure or service according a claims administrator and providers managed care contract.
Fee splitting: Unethical sharing of a fee with another physician Unethical sharing of a fee with another doctor based on services other than medical procedures and services performed like referring a patient.
Feedback: communication response.
Felony: A serious crime with a penalty of death or imprisonment.
Ferrous: iron containing.
Fetid: bad odor.
Field: A computer record's specific data element.
File: Group of records with similar information, often arranged in alphabetical or numerical order.
First morning specimen: First voided urine upon arising.
Fiscal: Pertaining to financial matters.
Fixative: Substance used to make fixed, preserved or firm in lab specimens or to maintain stability during transport.
Floppy disk: magnetic disks with a magnetic oxide coating over a thin plastic piece and used as a storage medium.
Fluoroscope: Device used to project an x-ray image for visual examination on a special screen.
Fluoroscopy: Visualization of internal body structures using a fluoroscope that often requires the use of a contrast medium.
Food and Drug Administration (FDA): The official federal agency responsible for the regulation of food, drugs, cosmetics

and medical devices and is part of the US Department of Health and Human Services.

Frenulum linguae: A mucous membrane making a longitudinal fold connecting the floor of the mouth to the underside of the tongue.

Gag reflex: When the glottis closes and constriction of its associated musculature responds to stimulation of the posterior pharynx by an object or substance in that area.

Gelatin culture: A culture of bacteria on a gelatin medium like agar.

Gender bias: Indicative of a specific gender with a type of language used.

Gender neutral: unable to determine when a gender is unable to be determined in a language.

Gene therapy: Replacement of a defective gene with a good gene to correct medical conditions.

Generalized: Widespread throughout the body.

Generic name: The common name for a drug such as aspirin.

Gerontology: Study of the effects of age and age-related diseases.

Glucosuria/glycosuria: glucose (sugar) present in urine,

Granulocyte: WBC that has granules in its cytoplasm.

Grievance: Real or imaginary wrong for the complaint.

Gross annual wage: whole salary before withholdings and taxes are taken out

Grounded: An electrical current or circuit connected with the ground through a solid connection or conductor.

Group practice: A practice of at least three doctors to share expenses.

Guardian ad litem: guardian ad litem; Court-appointed guardian to make decisions for a minor or unborn child in litigation.

Gynecology: The study of diseases and disorders of the female reproductive system.

Habituation: emotional dependence from repeated use of a drug.

Halo effect: A white surrounding line of light appearing around light possibly an indication of an eye disorder such as glaucoma.

Handbreadth: Use of a hand to measure distance on a patient for injection purposes.
Header: The top half of the transaction screen that accepts totals from each transaction.
Health maintenance organization (HMO): a company that provides comprehensive health care to an enrolled group of people at a fixed price.
Hemocytometer: Instrument for counting red and white blood cells.
Hematoma: Bruise
Hematopoiesis: Forming of blood cells.
Hematuria: blood in urine.
Hemiplegia: one side of body paralyzed.
Hemoglobin: Carries an iron containing pigment and oxygen which gives an RBC its color.
Hemolyzed: destruction of blood cells.
Hemoptysis: coughing blood.
Hemostatic: A drug medicine or blood component that stops bleeding.
Hernia: Protrusion of an organs wall.
High-power field (hpf): High power area of magnification of a microscope.
Histology: The study of the structure of a tissue.
Hives: Histamine induced peculiar raised patches of skin surrounded by redness; urticaria
Holistic, holistic: The human body viewed as a whole organism.
Homeopathy: Prevention and treatment of disease based on the idea that large doses of drugs that cause symptoms in healthy people will cure the same symptoms in small doses.
Homeostasis: balance of the human body.
Homophones: Words with different meanings that are spelled alike.
Honorarium: small payment. (i.e for a speech)
Hospice: Place for those with less than six months to live.
Hydrogenation: Process of changing unsaturated fat by adding hydrogen to become a solid saturated fat.
Hyfrecators: small electrocautery units that release heat for minor surgery.

Hypertension: High blood pressure.
Hypotension: Below normal blood pressure.
Hypothalamus: controls the autonomic nervous functions such as appetite, body temperature and sleep.
Idiosyncrasy: response to a drug or food abnormal to an individual.
Ileostomy: surgical opening in the small intestine for waste removal.
Immunity: disease resistance.
Inactive account: No transactions in a specified time period.
Incident report: A written formal report of an occurrence in a medical setting.
Incision: surgical cut.
Incontinent: unable to control excrement release.
Incubation: Period of time for microorgnanisms to grow or time period for a disease to develop after exposure.
Infarction: death of heart tissue.
Ingested: orally taken food or drink.
Inguinal: area between the hip and legs where flexion occurs.
Input: Information fed into the computer from a storage device, punched card or CRT.
Inspiration: To inhale.
Intermittent pulse: Occasionally skipping a heart beat.
Interrogation: Obtaining information by an authority asking a person who is often a witness.
Intravenous: To administer medication or fluid through a needle or catheter into a vein.
Invasive: entering the skin.
Kilograms: metric weight.
Labia: two folds of the female vaginal opening.
Laryngitis: larynx (voice box) inflammation causing temporary loss of voice
Lead(s): electrical connection or wires to sensors on the body when doing an EKG.
Ledger card: Record of charges, payments and current balance for each patient.
Legally binding: Contract that must be honored by law.
Leukemia: Cancerous condition of an increase in WBCs.

Leukocyte: A white blood cell.
Leukoplakia: Skin discoloration of white patches on mucous membranes that may become cancerous.
Liable: Responsible for compensation for a wrong.
Libel: False written statements about a person.
Licensure: Authorization to practice a profession after passing an examination.
Litigation: A court tried lawsuit.
Localized: Focal part of the body.
Low-power field (lpf): low power magnification of a microscopic field.
Lumen: open area within an object or organ.
Magnetic Ink Character Recognition (MICR): Characters and letters on the bottom of the check for routing to identify the bank number of an account.
Main memory: A part of the central processing unit that stores data and program instructions and does not perform any logical operations like computations and sorting.
Maintenance: The updating of records and files with current data including the functions ADD, CHANGE, DELETE, REACTIVATE.
Maker (of check): Payer.
Malaise: Discomfort associated with infection.
Malignant: Cancerous condition.
Malpractice: Negligence of a professional.
Mammogram: X-ray to detect breast cancer.
Managed care organization (MCO): A company that approves all non-emergency services, hospitalizations or tests before they are provided.
Master menu: A Controlling menu in a system of programs.
Matrix: format of a daily schedule.
Mature minor: One under age 18 and possessing an understanding of the nature and consequences of proposed treatment.
Mayo stand: Portable table or tray for surgical instruments to be placed during a procedure.
Media: broth, gelatin or agar to place microorganisms.

Medical asepsis: destroying organisms after they leave the body.
Medical emergency: life-threatening condition if not treated.
Medial ethics: moral behavior based on principles established for health care professionals.
Medial etiquette: Courtesy doctors extend to one another.
Medical privileges: doctor ability to admit a patient and practice medicine at a particular hospital.
Medically indigent: Person with no funds and no insurance coverage.
Medicare: Federal insurance program for health care for adults over 65 and disabled who qualify.
Medicinal: Substances like plants that provide a therapy.
Medulla oblongata: Brain part controlling the most important functions such as respiratory, cardiac and vasomotor centers of the brain.
Menstrual: Pertaining to a monthly uterine blood flow in women.
Menu: List to choose from to gain access to functions or programs.
Metastasize: A spreading of cancerous cells or tumors.
Metric system: A system of weight and measure that uses the decimal system.
Microbes: one-celled life form such as bacteria, algae, fungus and defined viruses.
Microcomputer: small, portable computer systems.
Microfiche: microfilm sheets.
Microprocessor: a small chip that processes date in a microcomputer.
Microscopic: Only visible under a microscope.
Minor: one under age 18.
Misdemeanor: A crime minor to a felony that carries a penalty of up to a year in prison and/or a fine.
Modified block: Letter writing style of the date, complimentary close and signature line beginning in the center with all other lines at the left margin.
Monitor: Screen to view input and output.

Monosaccharide: simple sugar unable to decompose further such as glucose or fructose.
Morale: Positive or negative emotional state of being with relation to work or work environment.
Morbidity rate: Number of diseased people in a certain population.
Mortality rate: death rate of a certain population.
Mouse: device controlling a pointer on a computer screen.
Myocardium: Muscle and fibrous tissue making up a heart wall.
Necrotic: death of tissue.
Negative: A culture failing to reveal a suspected organism.
Negligence: Failure to perform in a responsible manner one is obligated to do.
Negotiable: Transferring money to someone else through an endorsement on a check.
Neuroses: A condition when judgment is impaired by mild emotional disturbances.
No-show: Patient's absence from an appointment without notifying the physician's personnel.
Non-invasive procedure: When the body or skin is not entered into.
Nonparticipating provider: A physician's office that does not accept an allowable charge as the full fee for care.
Norm: Standard
Nosocomial infection: Infected in the hospital from one patient or person to another.
Nuclear medicine: Medical discipline involving the treatment of disease using radioactive isotopes.
Nutrient(s): Food or substance to supply necessary elements for a body's metabolism.
Obesity: 20% over the average weight of a person based on age, sex or height.
Obstructive lung disease: characterized by increased residual volume and slow expiratory rate.
Occult: Hidden.
Occult blood: Blood that can only be seen with a testing device such as Multistix.
Occurrence: abnormal event or incident.

Oliguria: Reduced urine production.
On-line: A computer's ability to access records; changes are made as the program specifies.
Open-ended questions: Questions requiring explanation.
Opportunistic infections: infections resulting from a reduced immune system such as pneumonia from AIDS.
Orifice: body opening.
Orthopnea: When breathing is easier sitting rather than lying.
Output: Computer generated information.
Outpatient: A patient who does not stay overnight for treatment. Also called "23 hour hold" or ambulatory.
Outstanding deposits: unprocessed checks deposited in an account.
Overbooking: scheduling multiple patients in the same time slot. Also called double or triple booking.
Override: A computers default field is replaced by an entry.
Oxyhemogiobin: Component of arterial blood that is a combination of oxygen and hemoglobin and carries oxygen to body tissues.
Pacemaker: Sinoatrial node of the heart or the artificial equipment used when the natural pacemaker fails.
Palpatory method: Using sense of touch to determine.
PAP smear: Papanicolaou test for cytology testing for early detection of cervical and vaginal cancer cells.
Parasites: An organism living within another organism.
Parenteral: Route for medication other than the alimentary canal (oral or rectal) such as subcutaneous, intravenous and intramuscular.
Participating provider: A physician's office who accepts an assignment for an insurance plan and paid directly by the plan.
Passcode: Pertaining to USER-ID, containing a field with up to six characters.
Password: A word or phrase that allows access or entry to a program.
Pasteurization: The process of destroying bacteria when heated to a particular temperature substance such as milk or cheese.
Pathogens: microorganisms that produce disease.
Pathologic: Relating to a condition of disease or injury.

Payee: receiving person or company to whom the amount on the check is payable.
Payer: person who signs a check to release money.
Pediatrics: The branch of medicine involving children.
Peer Review Organization (PRO): Professional organization to review a physician's conduct.
Perfusion: To supply an organ or tissues with oxygen and nutrients by injecting fluid or blood into an artery.
Physiatrist: a doctor who specializes in physical medicine and rehabilitation.
Plaintiff: A group or person who brings an action into litigation.
Postdate: When a future date on a check is written and the then signed.
Post transactions: In medical computers, batch transactions copied from daily files to files that are month to date.
Pre-register: When patient information is given to a medical assistant or secretary over the telephone prior to admission to a health care facility or insurer for prior approval; or it may be done prior to the patient's visit.
Preauthorization: a requirement of Medicare and insurance companies to obtain prior approval for procedures performed in order to receive reimbursement.
Precedent: law established in a prior case.
Predisposes: tendency for a certain condition or disease to develop.
Premium: amount to be paid for insurance coverage.
Prepaid plan: managed care plan where a group of healthcare providers have a contractual agreement to provide services to subscribers on a negotiated fee-for-service or captivated basis.
Procedure manual: A collection of day to day processes in an office or facility.
Production analysis: A percentage analysis report of activity in each CPT code.
Prognosis: prediction for an outcome of a disease.
Prompt: A cue or the next action to be taken on a screen that is a word or phrase.
Prophylaxis: preventing disease.

Proprietary hospital: A for-profit hospital.
Prosthesis: A body part that is artificial.
Protocol: Standard way of performing tasks.
Proximate cause: direct cause.
Psychoses: A severe mental disorder where there is loss of contact with reality evidenced by delusions.
Public duty: A doctor's responsibility to report cases of communicable diseases and abuses and to provide birth and death certificates.
Puerperal sepsis: childbed fever
Pulmonary volume tests: Under constant conditions, the patient makes extreme inhalations and exhalations and the amount of gas inhaled or exhaled is recorded.
Pulse deficit: A difference between the two pulses of the apical and radial pulse sites.
Pulse pressure: When the top and bottom number of a blood pressure reading is subtracted with systolic and diastolic.
Pure culture: A culture of an uncontaminated form of microorganism.
Pyrexia: Abnormally high body temperature; fever.
Quality assurance program (QAP): A program that hospitals and medical practices use to evaluate their services against with the accepted standards.
Reactivate: To change a flag on a record to regain its accessibility.
Reconciliation (of bank statement): adjusting one's banking records against a bank statement so both are in agreement.
Reflecting: Mirroring by repeating words back in a conversation.
Refractometer: Device to measure specific gravity of urine.
Renal colic: Pain in kidneys often due to kidney stones.
Repolarization: Return to polarization and rest from a depolarized state.
Res ipsa loquitur: Latin for "The thing speaks for itself." A doctrine of negligence law.
Reservoir: Source of infection.
Respondeat superior: Latin for "Let the master answer." The physician/employer is responsible for his employee's actions.

Restating: Using different terms to say what the patient had previously said.

Return through: When the return key can be repeatedly pressed after a screen display of a list of fields and one or more fields have either no data or have default data supplied.

Rider: A documented exception to an insurance contract that expands, decreases or modifies coverage of an insurance policy.

Right justified: When data is placed in the field and the most right positions are filled.

Rule of discovery: The statute of limitations begins at the time the injury is discovered or should have been is known by the patient.

Scrub assistant: A sterile assistant responsible for passing instruments, sponges or swabs bodily fluids from the operative site, retracts incisions and cuts sutures.

Settle: Determining the outcome of a case outside the courtroom.

Signee: Person who signs document.

Slander: Malicious and false spoken words about another.

Smears: A spread of bacteria on a microscopic slide or culture medium.

Smear fixation: To make a smear adhere to a glass slide by a fixative or heat.

Software: program

Solo practice: A single physician's business.

Solvent: Having money sufficient enough to pay debts.

Specific gravity (S.G): Comparison of the weight of a substance to an equal volume of water.

Specific time: Scheduling a time slot to one person.

Specimen(s): A sample part of something to show the quality or condition of it.

Speculum: Instrument for examining canals and body orifices.

Sputum: Substance from coughing or clearing of the bronchi sometimes used to discover possible causative agents of respiratory disease.

Squamous epithelial cells: Flat scale like cells attached at the edges that line the bladder visible under a microscope.
Standard of care: The ordinary skill and care that is commonly used by other medical practitioners when caring for patients.
Standardization: Test made to document a machine's compliance with the international agreement.
Statute of limitations: Maximum time allowed set by federal and state governments during which specific legal actions can be brought forward.
Sterile: A condition when all microorganisms and spores have been destroyed Sterile field
Stereile Field: An area prepared with sterile drapes for surgery that covers non-sterile areas.
Stool: Feces or bowel movement.
Stop payment: When the maker of a check writes to the bank not to honor the payment of a check for a charge of this service.
Sublingual: Under the tongue.
Subnormal: A temperature that is abnormally low.
Subpoena: Court order for a person or document to appear in court.
Superbill: Billing and insurance processing record. Also known as an encounter form or a charge slip.
Suppuration: Pus formation form infection.
Surgical asepsis: Technique for the maintenance of a sterile environment.
Symptom(s): An objective or subjective change in the body perceived by the patient that indicates a disorder..
Syncope: fainting
Syphilis: A venereal disease that is infectious and chronic with lesions and can affect many organs. Antibiotics are used to treat it.
Systemic: Relating to the entirety of a body.
Systole: Cardiac cycle period when the atria and ventricles contract and eject blood out of the heart.
Terminal digit filing: Filing medical records based on the last digits of the ID number.
Terminal disease: A disease expected to end in death.

Third party payer(s): Someone other than the patient who pays the patient's bills such as an insurance company.

Third-party check: check written to one person for payment and given to someone else for payment (the third payee).

Tidal volume: Total volume of air inspired and expired in one normal respiratory cycle.

Tinnitus: Condition of ringing in the ears.

Tort: Harmful act committed against a person or property.

Toxicity: The extent to which a substance is poisonous.

Tracing: Recording.

Transcription: Typing a sound recorded medical record.

Triage: Determination of thepriori9ty for handling patients with severe conditions or injuries.

Turbidity: Cloudiness in appearance.

Two hour postprandial: Length of time being two hours after eating a meal.

Tympanic membrane: Eardrum

United States Pharmacopeia-National Formulary (USP-NF): A drug book listing all official drugs in North America

Untoward effect: Undesirable side effect of a medication.

Urinary meatus: Orifice from the urethra to the outside of the body.

Urinary retention: Unable to release urine out of the body.

Urinometer: Device to measure specific gravity of urine.

Urticaria: Hives

Usual, customary and reasonable (UCR): A standard of fees charged by a majority of physicians for the same service and at a reasonable fee a patient might expect to pay. It is used to determine medical benefits.

Void: Urinate

Warrant: Written non-negotiable evidence of a debt to a person which can then be used to collect the money.

Wave: Flexible scheduling where all patients arrive at the beginning of the hour they are scheduled and each hour is divided into segments of time.

X-rays: Electromagnetic radiation of shorter wavelength than light rays that are visible and able to pass through opaque bodies.

BIBLIOGRAPHY

Fremgen, B.F. (1998). Essentials of Medical Assisting Administrative and Clinical Competencies. Upper Saddle River, NJ: Brady/Prentice Hall.

Beebe, M., Dalton, J.A., Duffy, C, Esproncoda, M., Evans, D.D., Friedman, R. et al. (Eds.). (2004) Current Procedural Terminology CPT 2005. American Medical Association: AMA Press.

Hart, A.C., Hopkins, C.A., Ford, B. (Eds.). (2005). 2006 ICD-9-CM Professional for physicians volumes 1&2 International Classification of Diseases 9th Revision Clinical Modification Sixth Edition. USA: Ingenix Inc.

American Psychological Association (2001). Publication Manual of the American Psychological Association, fifth edition. Washington DC: American Psychological Association.

The book Medical Assistant Handbook 5th edition (2004).

Hosley, J.B., Molle-Matthews, E.A. (1999). Lippincott's Pocket Guide to Medical Assisting. Philadelphia, PA: Lippincott Williams & Wilkins.

Christensen, B.L.& Kockrow, E.O. (2003). Foundations of Nursing. St. Louis, Missouri: Mosby.

Williams, L.S. & Hopper, P.D. (2003).
Understanding Medical Surgical Nursing.
Philadelphia, PA: F.A. Davis Company.

Bowden, B.S. & Bowden, J. (2002).
An Illustrated Atlas of the Skeletal Muscles.
Englewood, CO:
Morton Publishing Company.

Gylys, B.A., Wedding, M.E. (2005).
Medical Terminology Systems
A Body Systems Approach Fifth edition.
Philadelphia, PA: F.A. Davis Company.

Stapleton, E.R., Aufderheide, T.P.,
Hazinski, M.F., Cummins, R.O. (Eds.).
(2001). BLS for Healthcare Providers.
American Heart Association.

Venes, D. (ed.), (2005). Edition 20 Illustrated
in Full Color Taber's Cyclopedic Medical
Dictionary. Philadelphia, PA:
FA. Davis Company.

Duncan, C.H. (1990). College
Keyboarding/Typewriting Complete Course.
Cincinnati, OH: South-Western Publishing Co.

Mader, S.S. (2005). Understanding Human
Anatomy & Physiology, Fifth Edition.
New York, NY: McGraw Hill Higher
Education.

Gillogly, B. (1997). Skills and Techniques
For The New Nursing Assistant 2000 4th Edition.
Cypress, CA: Medcom.

Chameides, L., (ed.), (2002). Heartsaver First Aid.
Dallas, TX: American Heart Association.

Garza, D., and Becan-McBride, K. (2002).
Phlebotomy Handbook
Blood Collection Essentials.
Upper Saddle River, NJ:
Pearson Education, Inc.

Venes, D. (2001). Taber's Cyclopedic
Medical Dictionary.
Philadelphia, PA: F.A. Davis Company.

NCCLS: Procedures for the Collection of
Diagnostic Blood Specimens by Venipuncture;
Approved Standard – Fifth Edition; H3-A5,
Vol. 18, No.7; December 2003.

Ogden, S.J. (2003). Calculation of Drug Dosages.
St. Louis. Missouri: Mosby.

Saladin, K.S. (2001). Anatomy & Physiology
The Unity Of Form And Function-Second Edition.
New York, NY: McGraw-Hill.

Fleisher, G.R., Ludwig, S., Hentretig, F.M.,
Ruddy, R.M., Silverman, B.K. (eds.), (2000).
Textbook of Pediatric Emergency Medicine.
Philadelphia, PA: Lippincott Williams & Wilkins.

Behrman, R.E., Kliegman, R.M., Jenson, H.B. (2004).
Nelson Textbook Of Pediatrics, 17th Edition.
Philadelphia, PA: Saunders.

Pendergraph, G.E., Pendergraph, C.B. (1998).
Handbook Of Phlebotomy And Patient Service Techniques,
Fourth Edition. Baltimore, Maryland: Williams & Wilkins.

Green, C., Branson, C., Virgin, P. (1993).
American Red Cross Foundations For Caregiving.
Boston, MA: Mosby.

http://www.consumerfreedom.com

Giddens, J.F., Langford, R.W. (2004). Mosby's Nursing PDQ.
St. Louis, Missouri: Mosby.

www.ingramcontent.com/pod-product-compliance
Lightning Source LLC
Chambersburg PA
CBHW030755180526
45163CB00003B/1032